Be Pregnant

AN ILLUSTRATED COMPANION
FOR MOMS-TO-BE

Eugenia Viti

VORACIOUS

LITTLE, BROWN AND COMPANY

NEW YORK   BOSTON   LONDON

The Journey

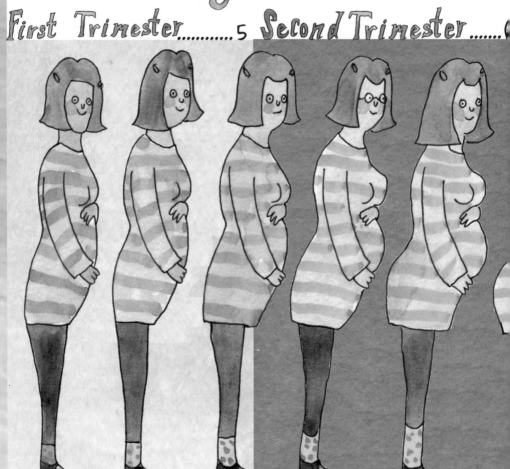

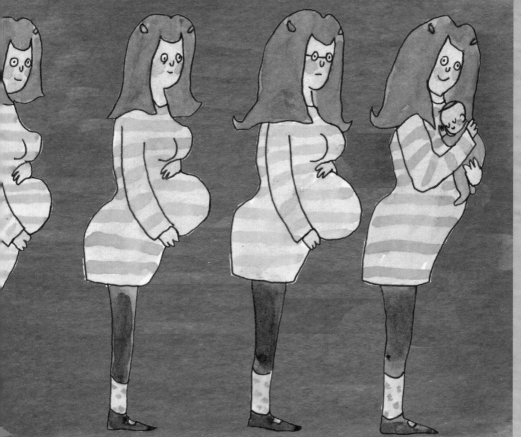

Voracious / Little, Brown and Company
Hachette Book Group
1290 Avenue of the Americas, New York, NY 10104
littlebrown.com

First Edition: March 2022

Voracious is an imprint of Little, Brown and Company, a division of Hachette Book Group, Inc. The Voracious name and logo are trademarks of Hachette Book Group, Inc.

The publisher is not responsible for websites (or their content) that are not owned by the publisher.

The Hachette Speakers Bureau provides a wide range of authors for speaking events. To find out more, go to hachettespeakersbureau.com or call (866) 376-6591.

Artwork by Eugenia Viti

ISBN 9780316628457
LCCN 2021939652

10 9 8 7 6 5 4 3 2 1

IM

Printed in China

IF PREGNANCY WAS A DRUG

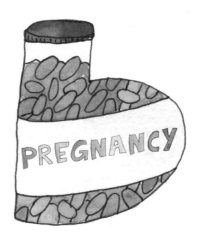

SIDE EFFECTS MAY INCLUDE: VOMITING, MISSED PERIOD, HEMORRHOIDS, DIABETES, EXHAUSTION, DIZZINESS, FREQUENT URINATION, MOOD SWINGS, SWOLLEN BREASTS, CRAVINGS, FATIGUE, FREQUENT DOCTOR VISITS, TROUBLE SLEEPING, WEIGHT GAIN, INSOMNIA, BLOATING, CRAMPING, LIGHT SPOTTING, UNSOLICITED ADVICE, INTRUSIVE QUESTIONS, UNSEEMLY JUDGMENT FROM OTHERS, CONSTIPATION, HEADACHES, GROWING BELLY, BRAXTON HICKS, URGE TO CLEAN, URGE TO NEST, GENERAL WORRY, SKIN CHANGES, DENTAL ISSUES, VAGINAL DISCHARGE, URINARY TRACT INFECTIONS, EXPANDING BELLY, FOOD AVERSIONS, NASAL CONGESTION, RESTLESS LEGS, PEEING ON SELF, LEG CRAMPS, DEBILITATING PAIN, DIARRHEA, SWOLLEN FEET AND ANKLES AND FINGERS, SHORTNESS OF BREATH, DEATH, BUT MOSTLY, CREATING LIFE AND LOVE.

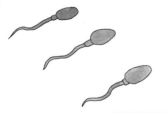

LIKE A FRIEND WHO'S BEEN THERE BEFORE

THIS BOOK IS MEANT TO ACCOMPANY A PREGNANT WOMAN THROUGH PREGNANCY. IT HAS SOME TIPS AND TRICKS AND IDEAS FOR HOW TO MAKE THE BEST OF IT, BUT IT'S NOT MEANT TO SHAME OR TELL YOU YOU'RE DOING IT WRONG.

WHILE PLENTY OF RESEARCH WENT INTO THIS BOOK, IT'S NOT WRITTEN BY A DOCTOR (OR EVEN APPROVED BY ONE!) SO WE'RE KEEPING THE FACTS TO THE POINT. AND AS MANY A MOM WILL TELL YOU, LOTS OF THE "GO-TO ADVICE" CHANGES OVER TIME.

MY PERSPECTIVE IS THAT IT'S NICE TO HAVE A COMPANION WHEN YOU GO ON TRIPS. AND PREGNANCY IS VERY MUCH LIKE A TRIP—YOU ARE CARRYING IMPORTANT CARGO, YOU ARE GOING TO A DESTINATION (BABYLAND), AND YOU WILL HAVE MANY NEW EXPERIENCES ALONG THE WAY. THIS BOOK IS A MIXTAPE, NOT A COMPASS, SO SIT BACK, RELAX, AND ENJOY WHEREVER THE JOURNEY LEADS YOU.

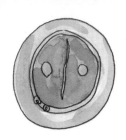
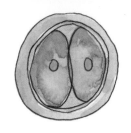
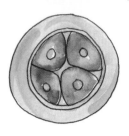

WHAT IS IT REALLY LIKE?

THIS BOOK WILL REVIEW EACH TRIMESTER'S EXCITING MOMENTS AND HARDSHIPS, COMMON MILESTONES, AND EXAMPLES OF "SOMETHING THAT MAY HAPPEN...". THIS BOOK ALSO INCLUDES INFORMATION ON LABOR AND BIRTH, AS WELL AS THE FOURTH TRIMESTER (THE FIRST THREE MONTHS AFTER THE BABY IS BORN). TAKE WHAT YOU WANT AND LAUGH AT THE REST.

THE APPROACH HERE IS "GLASS HALF FULL." THERE ARE ALREADY ENOUGH DOOMSDAY PRECAUTIONARY TALES OUT THERE FOR ALL THE PREGNANT WOMEN IN THE WORLD THREE TIMES OVER.

AND FINALLY, PREGNANCY IS EXPERIENCED IN MANY DIFFERENT WAYS. THERE IS LITERALLY NO ONE WAY TO BE PREGNANT. I TRIED TO INCLUDE MANY PERSPECTIVES, BUT THERE'S ONLY SO MUCH YOU CAN READ BEFORE THE BABY GETS HERE.

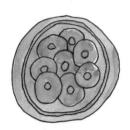
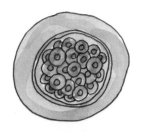
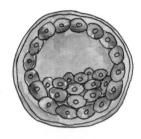

Milestones

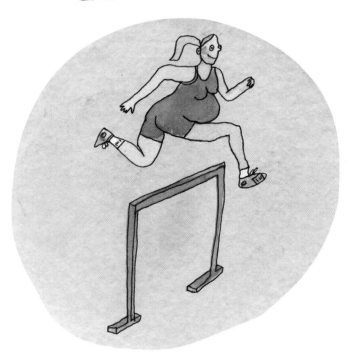

PREGNANCY IS FULL OF MILESTONES. THEY MAY FEEL LIKE HURDLES JUMPED IN A 40*-WEEK-LONG MARATHON. THE MILESTONES TAKE EFFORT, THEY ARE EXCITING TO CLEAR, AND RELIEF WASHES OVER YOU WHEN YOU FINALLY CROSS SOME. LIKE A FILTER ON A CAMERA, SOME OF THESE MOMENTS CAN ALSO ADD A NEW LAYER TO DAILY LIFE, MAKING PARTS OF PREGNANCY (DARE I SAY IT?) FUN. SOME EXAMPLES INCLUDE: THE FIRST PREGNANCY TEST, THE 20-WEEK ULTRASOUND, TELLING YOUR BOSS, BABY FLIPPING, AND MORE. LOOK OUT FOR THE HURDLE JUMPER ABOVE FOR MILESTONE PAGES THROUGHOUT THIS BOOK.

*PLUS OR MINUS A FEW WEEKS

First Trimester

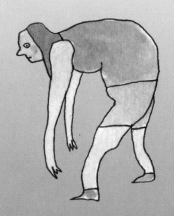

SHHH, IT'S A SECRET (?)

THE FIRST MONTH

SINCE IT'S BASICALLY IMPOSSIBLE TO KNOW IF YOU'RE PREGNANT THE FIRST MONTH, MANY PEOPLE WILL ACCIDENTALLY TAKE PART IN A FEW ACTIVITIES (OR A FEW TOO MANY DRINKS) THAT ARE NOT RECOMMENDED FOR PREGNANCY.

GARDENING: UNLIKE MOST OF THESE EXAMPLES, THERE AREN'T HORDES OF PEOPLE OUT THERE TELLING PREGNANT WOMEN NOT TO GARDEN, BUT IT'S TRUE: SINCE OUTDOOR CATS USE GARDENS AS BATHROOMS, GARDENING COULD LEAD TO THE SAME DANGERS AS CLEANING KITTY LITTER. BUT YOU CAN TAKE PRECAUTIONS, LIKE GARDENING WITH GLOVES AND HANDWASHING.

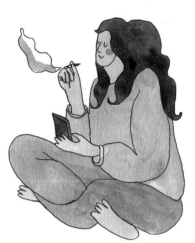

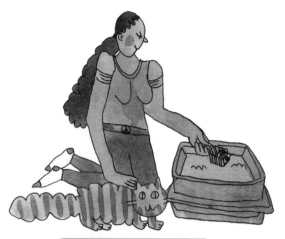

CLEANING KITTY LITTER

SMOKING

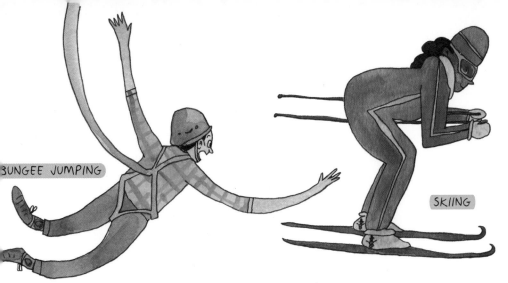

BUNGEE JUMPING

SKIING

EATING SUSHI: SOME TYPES OF SUSHI ARE ACTUALLY FINE! BUT YOU'LL WANT TO AVOID THAT PESKY (AND DELICIOUS) MERCURY-RICH FISH THAT'S OUT THERE.

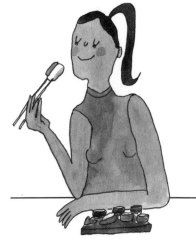

WHILE IT'S STILL A GOOD IDEA TO STOP THESE ACTIVITIES SHOULD YOU BE TRYING TO GET PREGNANT, THE PLACENTA HASN'T FORMED YET, SO YOUR BABY LIKELY WON'T BE AFFECTED. IF YOU'VE ALREADY DONE SOME OF THESE BEFORE YOU FOUND OUT YOU WERE PREGNANT, IT'S WATER UNDER THE BRIDGE.

DRINKING

7

At One Month

ALIEN SEAHORSE

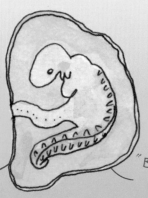

THE FETUS HAS RECENTLY IMPLANTED TO THE UTERINE WALL AND THE PLACENTA IS STARTING TO FORM.

"BABY" HAS GROWN FROM A FEW MICROSCOPIC CELLS TO A VISIBLY SMALL, TAILED CREATURE.

WEEKS 1-4

YOU MAY HAVE A HUNCH THAT YOU'RE PREGNANT, BUT MOST PEOPLE AREN'T SURE IN THE FIRST MONTH. SOME WOMEN START FEELING SYMPTOMS RIGHT AWAY, WHILE OTHERS FEEL EXACTLY THE SAME.

AVERAGE END-OF-MONTH SIZE: 0.3 IN (8 MM)

First-Trimester Feelings
KEEPING A SECRET

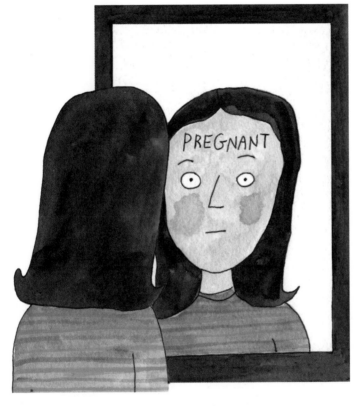

THE FIRST TRIMESTER CAN FEEL IMPERSONAL BECAUSE YOU'RE EXCITED THERE'S SOMEONE IN THERE, BUT YOU ARE SUPPOSED TO KEEP IT A SECRET IN CASE SOMETHING GOES WRONG. IT MIGHT FEEL UNFAIR THAT YOU HAVE TO KEEP THIS NEW DEVELOPMENT A SECRET AS THOUGH IT'S SHAMEFUL. DESPITE SOCIAL NORMS, YOU SHOULD DO WHATEVER FEELS RIGHT FOR YOU.

9

PREGNANCY POLARIZATION

THERE ARE LOTS OF PRECONCEIVED (PUN INTENDED) NOTIONS WHEN PEOPLE SEE THAT BUMP. IT'S LIKE YOU'RE EITHER THE PERFECT PREGNANT LADY OR THE OPPOSITE. EVEN WHEN PEOPLE ASK HOW YOU'RE DOING, AND YOU ARE POTENTIALLY IN GREATER AND GREATER PAIN EACH DAY, IT'S LIKE YOU ARE NOT ALLOWED TO SAY HOW YOU REALLY FEEL. JEEZ! NO ONE CAN TELL YOU HOW YOU SHOULD FEEL, NO MATTER WHETHER YOU HAVE A TINY BABY INSIDE YOU OR NOT! THERE IS NO WRONG WAY TO BE PREGNANT.

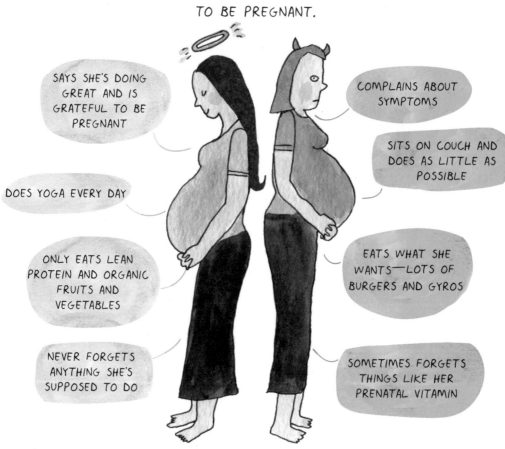

SAYS SHE'S DOING GREAT AND IS GRATEFUL TO BE PREGNANT

COMPLAINS ABOUT SYMPTOMS

SITS ON COUCH AND DOES AS LITTLE AS POSSIBLE

DOES YOGA EVERY DAY

ONLY EATS LEAN PROTEIN AND ORGANIC FRUITS AND VEGETABLES

EATS WHAT SHE WANTS—LOTS OF BURGERS AND GYROS

NEVER FORGETS ANYTHING SHE'S SUPPOSED TO DO

SOMETIMES FORGETS THINGS LIKE HER PRENATAL VITAMIN

AN AWESOME PREGNANT WOMAN   AN EQUALLY AWESOME PREGNANT WOMAN

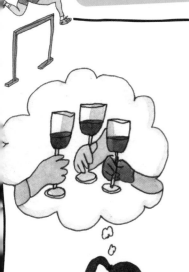

FINDING OUT

YOU MISS YOUR PERIOD BY ONE DAY AND DECIDE YOU SHOULD PROBABLY GET A PREGNANCY TEST BEFORE THAT WINE TASTING TOMORROW. SO YOU MAKE YOUR WAY TO THE LOCAL PHARMACY.

EVEN THOUGH YOU HAVE BEEN TRYING TO GET PREGNANT, THE THOUGHT OF BUYING A PREGNANCY TEST STILL MAKES YOU FEEL UNCOMFORTABLE. YOU REMEMBER THE LAST TIME YOU BOUGHT ONE WAS WHEN YOU WERE A TEEN AND YOU REALLY FELT SHAMED AND SCARED THEN.

NOW YOU'RE READY! IT SHOULDN'T BE THIS WAY, BUT YOU FEEL LIKE YOU ARE GOING TO BE JUDGED!

AT THE PHARMACY THERE ARE LIKE 45 PREGNANCY TESTS TO CHOOSE FROM. YOU STARE AT THE TESTS FOR TOO LONG TRYING TO FIGURE OUT WHICH ONE YOU SHOULD BUY. AFTER SOME TIME, YOU DECIDE TO GET THE STORE BRAND THAT COMES WITH THREE TESTS. YOU THINK, MAYBE IT'S THE BEST DEAL, BUT ACTUALLY YOU HAVE NO IDEA. WHY ARE THERE SO MANY? AREN'T THEY ALL THE SAME?

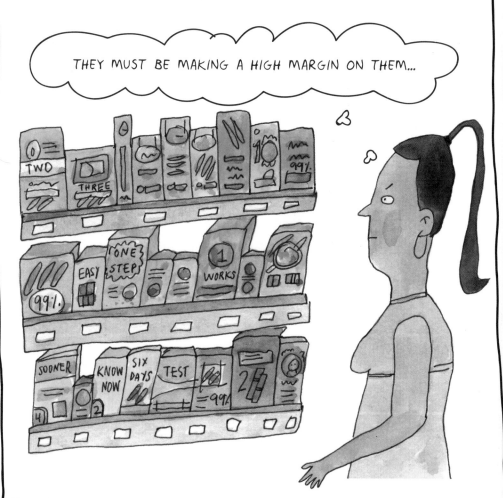

THEY MUST BE MAKING A HIGH MARGIN ON THEM...

YOU FEEL NERVOUS AS YOU WALK UP TO CHECK OUT. HOWEVER, YOU ARE ALSO THE QUEEN OF ACTING TOTALLY CONFIDENT—EVEN WHEN YOU ARE NOT FEELING IT. SO YOU WALK UP AS CONFIDENTLY AS YOU CAN WITH ONLY THE PREGNANCY TEST TO THE CASHIER.

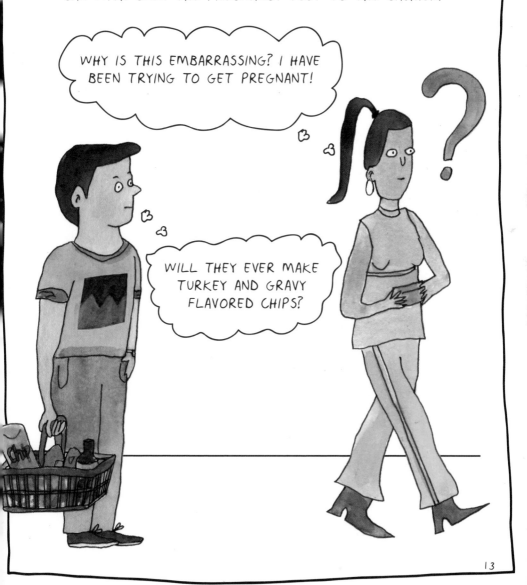

THE CHECKOUT LADY'S SMALL TALK SEEMS EXTRA KIND. YOU HAVE A GOOD INTERACTION WITH HER, AND YOU HAVE A GOOD FEELING ABOUT THE TEST.

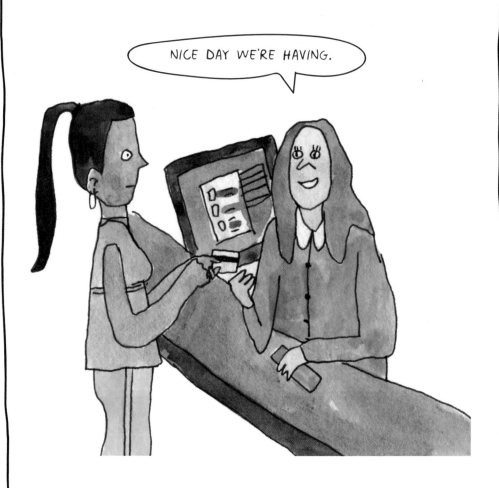

YOU GO HOME AND YOU PEE ON THE TEST AND SHOWER WHILE IT WORKS ITSELF OUT. WHILE IN THE SHOWER YOU PEEK OUT AND SEE THAT IT SHOWS TWO LINES.

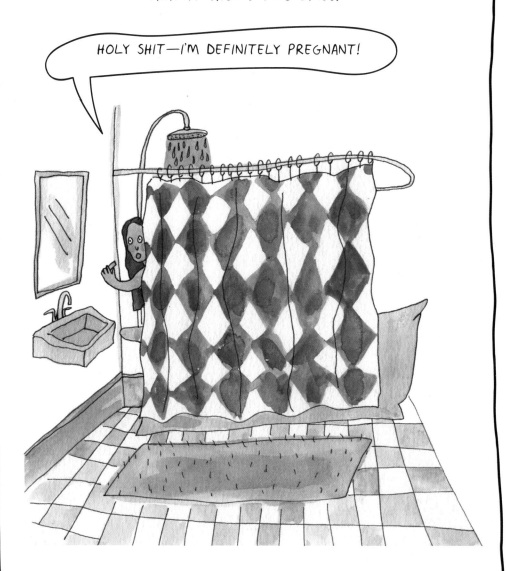

YOU PEE ON A SECOND STICK, AND IT'S ALSO POSITIVE. YOU HAVE A WORK CALL SOON, AND YOU ARE INTERNALLY FREAKING OUT. YOU TEXT YOUR PARTNER ABOUT IT AND THEN YOU TAKE YOUR WORK CALL AS IF NOTHING MAJOR HAS CHANGED IN YOUR LIFE JUST NOW.

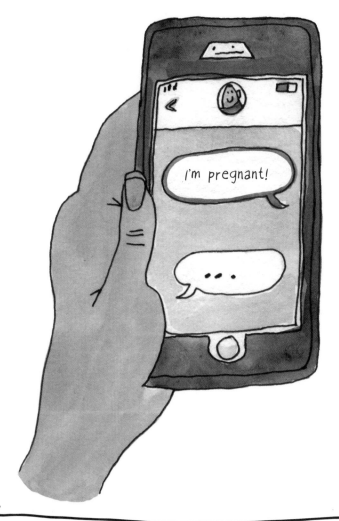

YOUR SIGNIFICANT OTHER COMES HOME A FEW HOURS LATER AND IS IN DISBELIEF. HE ASKS IF YOU'RE SURE YOU ARE PREGNANT AND SAYS THAT YOU SHOULD SCHEDULE AN APPOINTMENT WITH THE DOCTOR TO CONFIRM. YOU ARE ANNOYED AT HIS REACTION. YOU JUST TOOK TWO TESTS! BUT ALSO, MAYBE TEXT WASN'T THE BEST WAY OF TELLING HIM. IN THE END YOU BOTH LAUGH IT OFF.

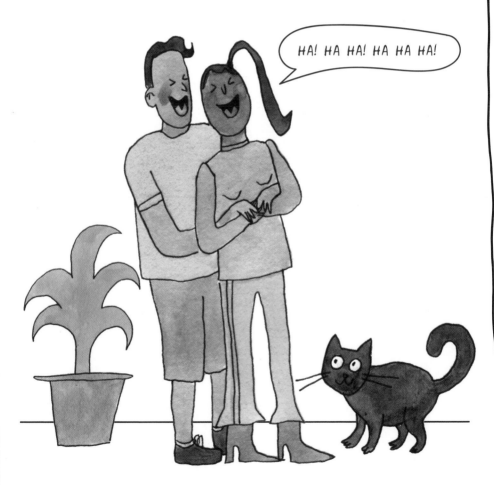

Midwife/Doctor/Doula

CHOOSING YOUR MEDICAL TEAM

ONCE YOU KNOW YOU'RE PREGNANT YOU CAN SCHEDULE YOUR FIRST DOCTOR APPOINTMENT, BUT YOU WON'T GO IN UNTIL YOU'RE ABOUT SIX TO EIGHT WEEKS ALONG. NOW IS A GOOD TIME TO START THINKING ABOUT YOUR BIRTH TEAM AND BIRTH LOCATION.

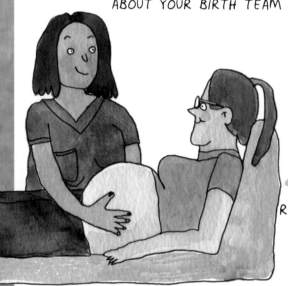

Midwife

GENERALLY RECOMMENDED WHEN:

- YOU'RE HEALTHY
- IT'S A SINGLETON (YES, THIS IS A REAL TERM FOR HAVING ONE BABY!)
- YOU'RE YOUNGER
- YOU WANT A MIDWIFE

A MIDWIFE IS A HEALTH PROFESSIONAL WHOSE MAIN FUNCTION IS HELPING HEALTHY WOMEN DURING LABOR, DELIVERY, AND POSTPARTUM.

THE STRANGE NAME COMES FROM OLD ENGLISH, MEANING "WITH WOMAN" OR SOMEONE WHO IS LITERALLY WITH A WOMAN DURING CHILDBIRTH. MIDWIVES ARE GENERALLY THOUGHT TO USE LESS INTRUSIVE METHODS AND TO BE ABLE TO GIVE MORE INDIVIDUALIZED ATTENTION TO THE PATIENT DURING LABOR.

18

Doctor

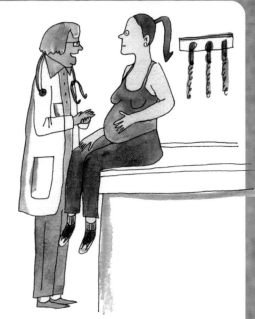

GENERALLY RECOMMENDED WHEN:

- YOU HAVE COMPLICATIONS
- IT'S MULTIPLES
- YOU'RE OLDER
- YOU WANT OR NEED A C-SECTION
- YOU WANT A DOCTOR

JUST LIKE MIDWIVES, AN OBSTETRICIAN-GYNECOLOGIST CAN TAKE CARE OF A PREGNANT WOMAN THROUGH PREGNANCY, BIRTH, AND POSTPARTUM. UNLIKE MIDWIVES, OB-GYNS ARE ABLE TO USE FORCEPS AND VACUUMS AS WELL AS OPERATE TO ASSIST DELIVERY.

Doula

WHAT'S THEIR DEAL?

ON TOP OF CHOOSING EITHER A MIDWIFE OR AN OB-GYN TO DELIVER YOUR BABY, YOU CAN HIRE A DOULA TO HELP AS WELL. MOST INSURANCE WON'T COVER DOULAS, WHICH IS A SHAME SINCE THEY TEND TO PROVIDE IMPORTANT SUPPORT. THE NEXT PAGE TELLS YOU MORE ABOUT WHAT DOULAS DO AND DON'T DO. (WOW, TRY SAYING THAT TEN TIMES FAST.)

Doula dos

- DO GENERALLY SUPPORT YOU IN WHAT YOU CHOOSE TO DO FOR THE BIRTH
- DO HELP YOU MAKE THE BEST DECISIONS FOR YOU THROUGH INFORMED CHOICES DURING THE BIRTH
- DO HELP CREATE A PEACEFUL AND CALM ATMOSPHERE (IF THAT'S WHAT YOU WANT!) DURING BIRTH
- DO HELP YOU THINK THROUGH A BIRTH PLAN IF YOU CHOOSE TO CREATE ONE (MORE ON THIS ON PAGES 132–134)
- DO HELP YOUR BIRTH BE THE BEST ONE IT CAN BE
- DO HELP SUPPORT YOUR PARTNER AS WELL DURING LABOR
- DO HELP YOU FEEL HEARD AND RESPECTED DURING YOUR BABY'S BIRTH

Doula don'ts

- DON'T SPEAK FOR YOU (THEY WILL ONLY HELP YOU ASK QUESTIONS)
- DON'T PUSH YOU TO GIVE BIRTH UNMEDICALLY (OR SOME OTHER WAY THAT YOU WOULDN'T WANT)
- DON'T REPLACE MEDICAL PROFESSIONALS

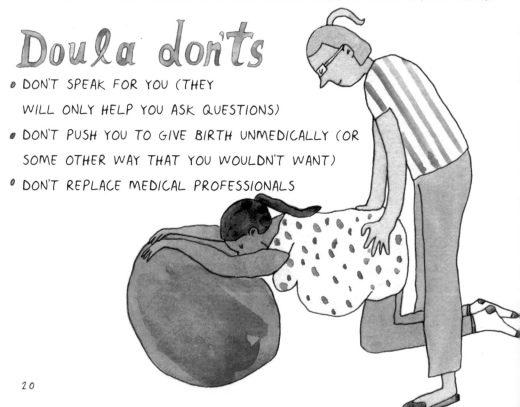

ALL KINDS OF PREGNANCIES

NO TWO PREGNANCIES ARE THE SAME—NOT EVEN FOR THE SAME WOMAN.
MANY START OFF WITH FACTORS THAT WILL CHANGE PREGNANCIES FROM
THE BEGINNING. SOME FACTORS CHANGE THE CARE YOU CHOOSE TO HAVE.

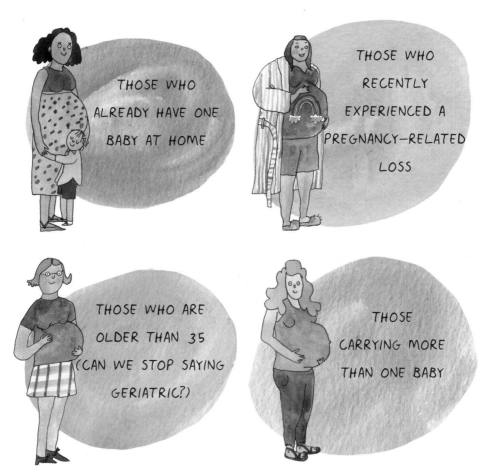

THOSE WHO
ALREADY HAVE ONE
BABY AT HOME

THOSE WHO
RECENTLY
EXPERIENCED A
PREGNANCY-RELATED
LOSS

THOSE WHO ARE
OLDER THAN 35
(CAN WE STOP SAYING
GERIATRIC?)

THOSE
CARRYING MORE
THAN ONE BABY

WHAT BRINGS US ALL TOGETHER IS THE MAGICAL JOURNEY OF
CREATING A LITERAL HUMAN INSIDE OF OURSELVES. WOMEN ARE AMAZING.

PRENATAL VISITS

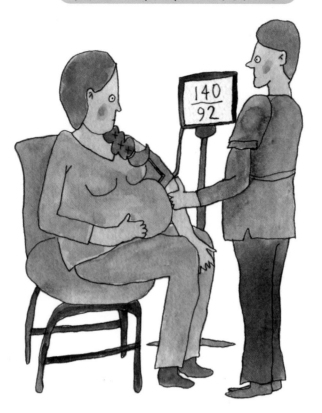

PART OF THE MIDWIFE'S OR OB-GYN'S ROLE WILL BE TO ADMINISTER YOUR PRENATAL PHYSICAL CHECKS ALONG WITH YOUR NURSES. THESE WILL LIKELY HAPPEN MONTHLY AT FIRST, THEN BIWEEKLY, THEN WEEKLY. IT'S HONESTLY A LOT OF APPOINTMENTS. HOWEVER, PRENATAL CARE IS SUPER IMPORTANT FOR DIAGNOSING VERY DANGEROUS CONDITIONS SO THAT PROPER STEPS CAN BE TAKEN TO KEEP MOM AND BABY HEALTHY. CONDITIONS LIKE PREECLAMPSIA AND GESTATIONAL DIABETES CAN BE VERY SERIOUS AND CAN GO ON UNDETECTED IF NOT FOR THESE CHECKS.

CHOOSING YOUR BIRTH LOCATION

GOES HAND IN HAND WITH CHOOSING A MIDWIFE OR OB-GYN

AT A HOSPITAL: THIS IS THE DEFAULT OPTION FOR MOST, WITH ABOUT 98% OF BIRTHS HAPPENING IN HOSPITALS. SOME THINGS TO CONSIDER WHEN CHOOSING A HOSPITAL:

- IS IT COVERED BY YOUR INSURANCE?
- IS IT CLOSE BY?
- WHAT LEVEL* NICU DOES IT HAVE?
- WHAT SORT OF STATISTICS CAN YOU FIND ON IT?
  (EXAMPLES: C-SECTION RATE, EPIDURAL RATE,
  PERCENT OF BABIES IN NICU)
- DOES IT FEEL RIGHT?

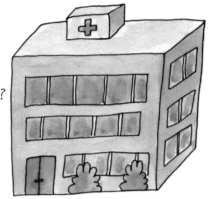

NOT AT A HOSPITAL: ALTHOUGH ONLY A SMALL PERCENTAGE OF BIRTHS HAPPEN EITHER AT HOME OR AT A BIRTHING CENTER, THE PERCENTAGE HAS INCREASED RECENTLY. LACK OF COVERAGE FROM INSURANCE IS ONE REASON WOMEN DO NOT CHOOSE THIS OPTION. ALSO, SOME STATES DON'T HAVE ENOUGH BIRTHING CENTERS TO REALLY CONSIDER IT AN OPTION. BIRTHING CENTERS TEND TO HAVE MORE COMFORTABLE FURNITURE AND BATHTUBS TO LABOR IN. HOWEVER, THEY LACK SOME GEAR THAT HOSPITALS HAVE FULL ACCESS TO (NICU OR OPERATING ROOM).

*THIS IS A STANDARDIZED RATING THAT INDICATES A HOSPITAL'S RESOURCES FOR TAKING CARE OF SICK BABIES AND THOSE BORN PREMATURELY.

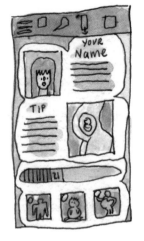

PREGNANCY APPS

YOUR MEDICAL TEAM SHOULD PROVIDE BASIC INFO, BUT MANY PEOPLE CHOOSE APPS TO TRACK BABY'S DAILY GROWTH AND DEVELOPMENT. WEIRD THING IS, MY APP SAID MY BABY WAS THE SIZE OF A TOMATO ONE WEEK, THEN THE SIZE OF A CUCUMBER THE NEXT! MUST BE A GIANT TOMATO.... PREGNANCY APPS ARE FUN TO MAKE FUN OF BUT, HEY, SOME OF THE INFO ON THERE IS REALLY INTERESTING.

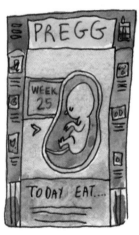

HOWEVER, IF YOU'RE NOT COMFORTABLE WITH AN APP OWNING AND POTENTIALLY MONETIZING YOUR AND YOUR OFFSPRING'S DATA, YOU CAN ALWAYS GOOGLE THE SAME INFO WHILE IN INCOGNITO MODE ON YOUR BROWSER. TO EACH THEIR OWN.

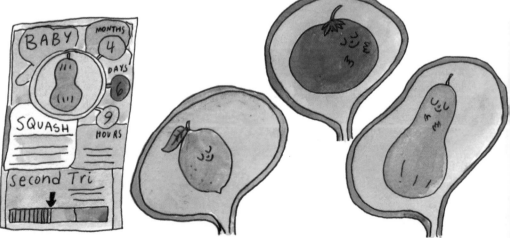

THERE IS NO HIDING FROM THE ALGORITHM

YOU AVOID GETTING A PREGNANCY APP, BUT WITH ALL YOUR GOOGLING YOU STILL START TO GET STRANGE ADS.

BUTT—ALTERING JEANS

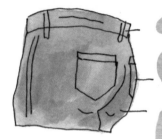

SQUEEZES YOUR FAT WAIST (RUDE!)

POCKETS THAT FLATTER—CAN'T THEY JUST BE POCKETS?

SAGGY ASS—LIFTING TECHNOLOGY—LEAVE MY ASS ALONE!

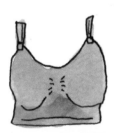

MATERNITY BRA OR TANK TOP?

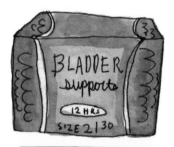

BLADDER supports
12 HRS
SIZE 2|30

PADS THAT ARE ACTUALLY JUST DIAPERS BUT MORE EXPENSIVE

WHY DOES IT SOMETIMES FEEL LIKE ADS TRY TO BULLY YOU INTO BUYING THEIR ITEMS? LET US LOVE OUR BUTTS IN PEACE AND SO FORTH.

The Body

SPEAKING OF BUTTS, LET'S TALK ABOUT THE BODY IN THE FIRST
TRIMESTER. THERE ARE TWO THINGS THAT INFAMOUSLY AFFECT THE BODY
RIGHT NOW. ONE IS FEELING NAUSEOUS. HOWEVER, JUST LIKE ALL ASPECTS
OF PREGNANCY, EVERYONE'S EXPERIENCE OF MORNING SICKNESS CAN VARY.
SOME PEOPLE DON'T FEEL ANY DIFFERENT AND CAN GET AWAY WITH
EATING EVERY COUPLE OF HOURS AND NEVER THROWING UP; FOR OTHERS,
NO MATTER WHAT THEY DO, THEY WILL THROW UP EVERY DAY. IF IT'S BAD,
DON'T HESITATE TO ASK YOUR DOCTOR ABOUT IT. THEY CAN HELP YOU OUT.

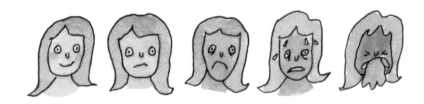

THE SECOND THING IS THE FATIGUE. THIS IS PRETTY REAL FOR MOST
PEOPLE, BUT AGAIN AFFECTS EVERYONE DIFFERENTLY. IF YOU CAN, GIVE
YOURSELF TIME TO RELAX AND SNACK.

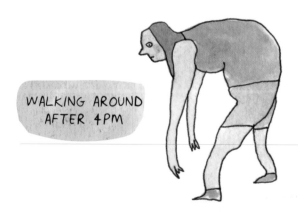

WALKING AROUND
AFTER 4PM

EVERYONE KNOWS ABOUT
THE NAUSEA...

BUT FEWER PEOPLE TALK ABOUT THE FACT THAT YOU MIGHT PUKE SO HARD THAT YOU PEE YOURSELF. SOMETIMES PREGNANCY IS SO HORRIBLE THAT IT BECOMES FUNNY, AND YOU JUST HAVE TO LAUGH ABOUT WETTING YOUR PANTS FOR THE THIRD DAY IN A ROW.

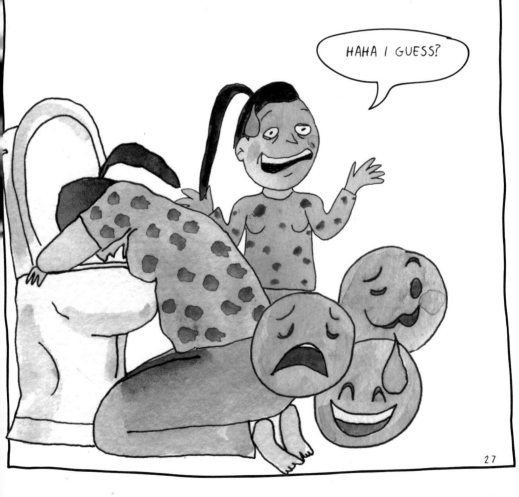

27

FIRST TRIMESTER: SUPERHERO

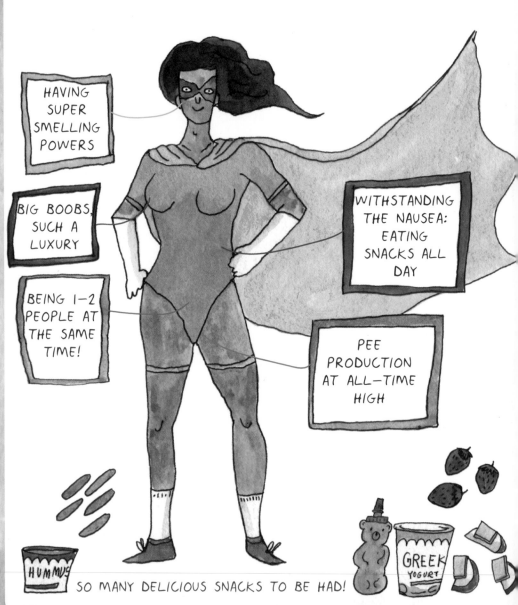

HAVING SUPER SMELLING POWERS

BIG BOOBS, SUCH A LUXURY

BEING 1-2 PEOPLE AT THE SAME TIME!

WITHSTANDING THE NAUSEA: EATING SNACKS ALL DAY

PEE PRODUCTION AT ALL-TIME HIGH

HUMMUS

GREEK YOGURT

SO MANY DELICIOUS SNACKS TO BE HAD!

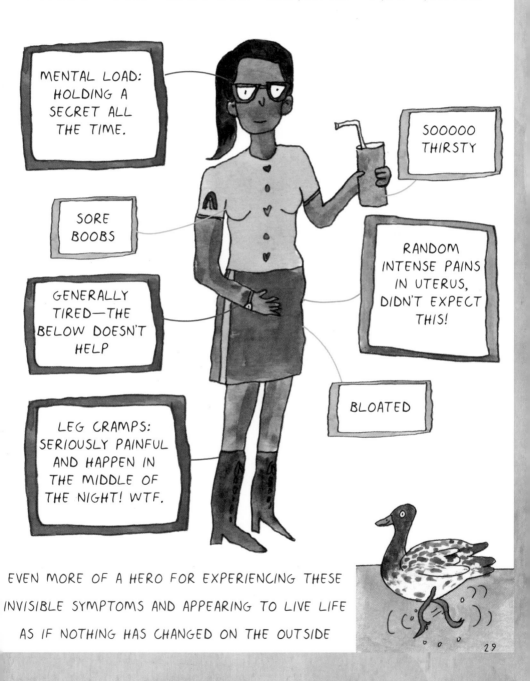

YOGA CLASS

YOU ARE STAYING ACTIVE DURING YOUR FIRST TRIMESTER OF PREGNANCY BY CONTINUING TO ATTEND YOUR WEEKLY YOGA CLASS. ONE DAY THE YOGA CLASS STARTS OFF NORMAL, BUT IT KEEPS GETTING HARDER AND HARDER.

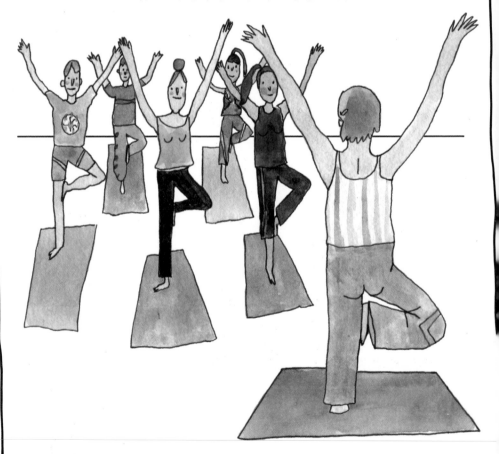

TOWARDS THE END OF THE CLASS THE TEACHER ASKS EVERYONE TO GO TO THE WALL AND PRACTICE DOING HANDSTANDS. THIS IS A MOVE THAT YOU HAVE NEVER DONE BEFORE. NORMALLY, YOU WOULDN'T SHY AWAY FROM SOMETHING NEW, BUT THIS TIME YOU FEEL SORT OF DIFFERENT.

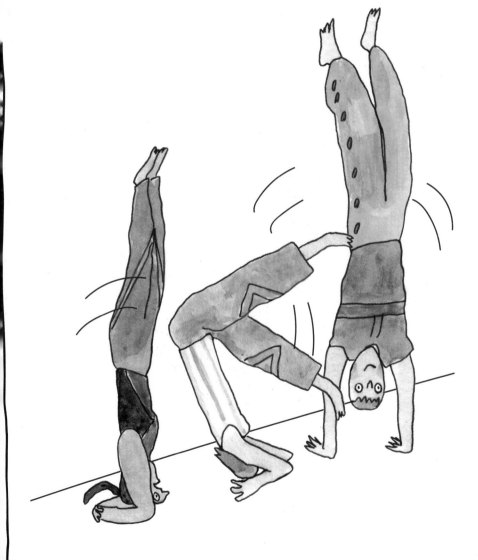

YOU STARE AS EVERYONE LINES UP AGAINST THE WALL AND STARTS KICKING INTO THE AIR AND DOING HANDSTANDS. YOU JUST DO NOT FEEL SAFE DOING THAT MOVE.

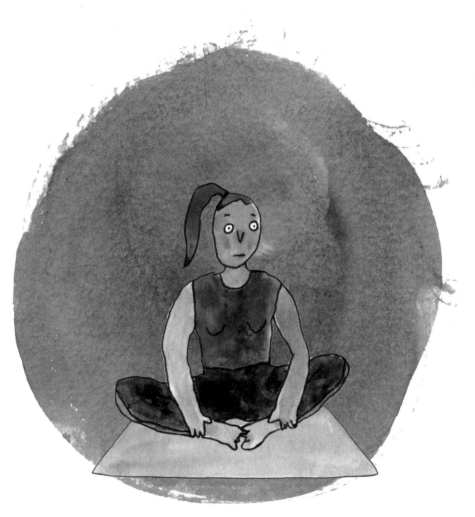

TWO PEOPLE OFFER YOU A SPOT ON THE WALL, BUT YOU JUST DON'T WANT TO TRY TO DO HANDSTANDS. YOU'VE NEVER BEEN AFRAID TO TRY A YOGA MOVE BEFORE, BUT SOMEHOW BEING PREGNANT MAKES SEEING ALL THOSE LEGS FLAILING AROUND IN SUCH CLOSE PROXIMITY... SCARY. YOU'RE NOT REALLY SURE WHY YOU FEEL THIS WAY, BUT MAYBE IT'S TO DO WITH FEELING CAUTIOUS ABOUT YOUR BODY AND BABY RIGHT NOW.

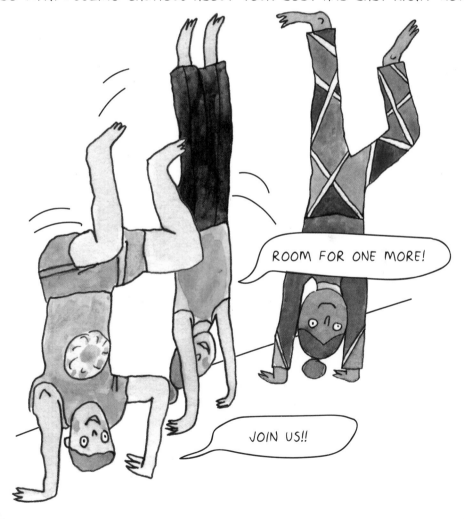

THE TEACHER COMES OVER TO WHERE YOU'RE SITTING AND OFFERS TO HELP YOU. YOU SORT OF WHISPER, "I'M AFRAID TO DO THAT." SHE IS TOTALLY OKAY WITH IT, BUT YOU FEEL LIKE CRYING. YOU FEEL THIS RUSH OF EMOTION, AS IF SOMETHING REALLY BAD HAS JUST HAPPENED—NOT SOMETHING AS SMALL AS SITTING OUT FROM A NEW MOVE DURING YOUR ELECTIVE ADULT YOGA CLASS. YOU ALMOST START CRYING, BUT YOU MANAGE TO JUST BREATHE AND RELAX AND KEEP STRETCHING.

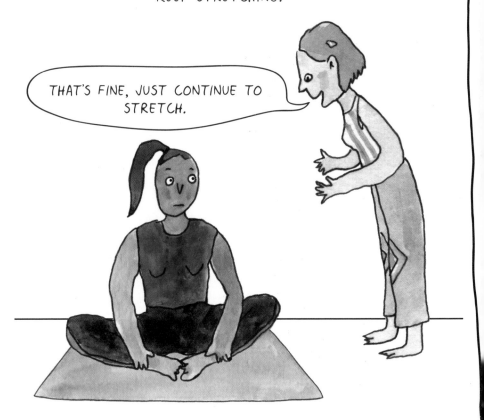

THE CLASS ENDS SOON AFTER THE HANDSTANDS, AND AS YOU HEAD HOME, YOU REFLECT ON THE EXPERIENCE. IT FELT LIKE YOU WERE IN JUNIOR HIGH GYM CLASS AND BEING TEASED BY YOUR CLASSMATES. WHAT A STRANGE FEELING TO HAVE AS A GROWN WOMAN. THEN YOU LOOK AT REDDIT, AND YOU SEE A REOCCURRING THEME: "TIC" OR "TODAY I CRIED." OF COURSE! YOUR HORMONES ARE CHANGING, JUST LIKE GOING THROUGH PUBERTY! IT'S HELPFUL TO SEE OTHERS GOING THROUGH SIMILAR EXPERIENCES, CRYING OVER THINGS THAT THEY NORMALLY WOULDN'T. YOU ARE RELIEVED YOU ARE NOT ALONE.

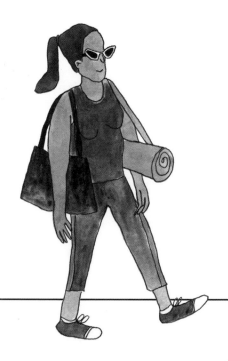

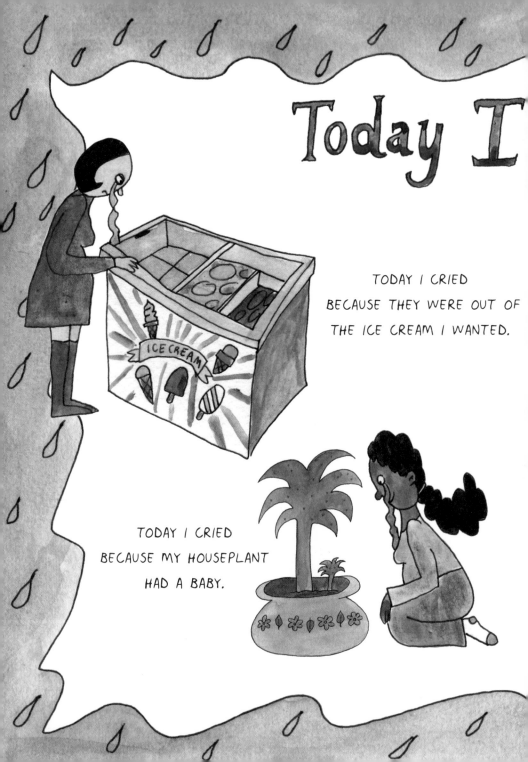

Today I

TODAY I CRIED
BECAUSE THEY WERE OUT OF
THE ICE CREAM I WANTED.

TODAY I CRIED
BECAUSE MY HOUSEPLANT
HAD A BABY.

Cried

TODAY I CRIED BECAUSE MY BRA WAS UNCOMFORTABLE.

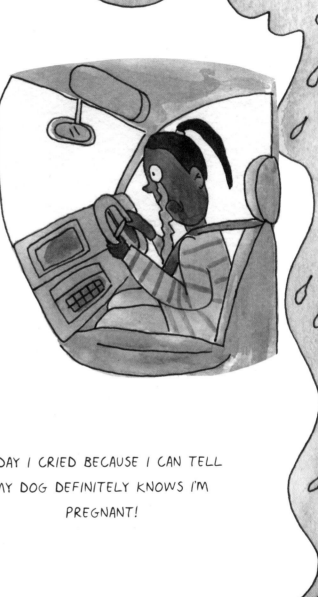

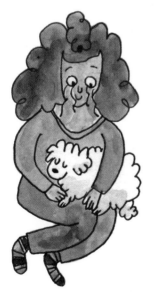

TODAY I CRIED BECAUSE I CAN TELL MY DOG DEFINITELY KNOWS I'M PREGNANT!

WET PANTIES

IT'S NOT SUPER CONVENIENT, BUT DURING PREGNANCY, PANTIES GET WET.*
WHAT IS CONVENIENT IS HAVING EXTRA UNDERWEAR ON HAND TO CHANGE
INTO. IF YOU WANT AND CAN, MAKE IT EASY AND BUY YOURSELF A COUPLE
NEW PACKS OF A SIZE LARGER THAN YOU NORMALLY WEAR. BIG COMFY
PANTIES ARE UNDERRATED ANYWAYS.

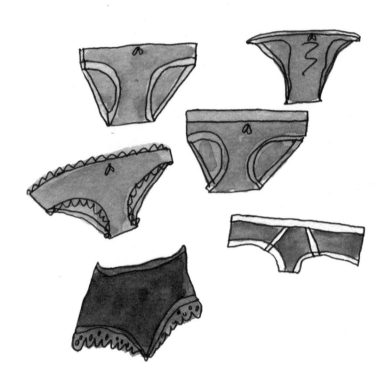

*WET FROM HEALTHY DISCHARGE

At Two Months

BELUGA WHALE

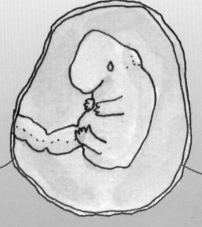

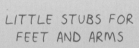
LITTLE STUBS FOR
FEET AND ARMS

THE HEART HAS
FORMED

WEEKS
5-8

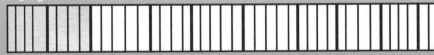

GREAT JOB GROWING THAT BABY. IT'S HARD WORK AND
YOU'RE NOT ALONE IF YOU'RE FEELING TIRED. YOU GOT THIS!

AVERAGE END-OF-MONTH SIZE: 0.63 IN (1.6 CM)

BEHAVIORAL CHANGES?

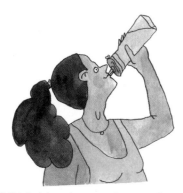

DRINKING SO MUCH MORE WATER.
DID YOU KNOW A PREGNANT
WOMAN'S BLOOD VOLUME CAN
INCREASE BY 50%?

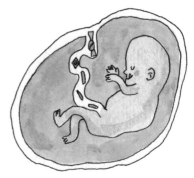

EATING DIFFERENTLY BECAUSE
YOU'RE PICTURING THE FETUS
EATING IT TOO.

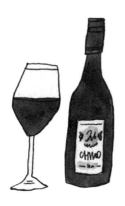

NO MORE ALCOHOL—OR
AT LEAST, NOT AS
MUCH.

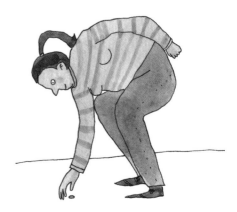

NO MORE EATING THINGS OFF
THE FLOOR.

FIRST DOCTOR APPOINTMENT

YOUR DOC WILL HAVE A MORE DETAILED (AND MEDICAL) LIST OF POTENTIAL CHANGES TO YOUR BEHAVIOR, BUT THREE MAIN THINGS WILL HAPPEN DURING YOUR FIRST APPOINTMENT:

PEE IN A CUP: THIS WILL CONTINUE FOR EACH APPOINTMENT AND GET HARDER AND HARDER TO DO! GOOD THING THEY INVENTED THOSE LITTLE HANDLES ON THE CUPS.

LAST PERIOD: THEY'LL ASK ABOUT IT, TO CALCULATE THE ESTIMATED DUE DATE. SINCE WOMEN DIFFER IN CYCLE LENGTH, THE ULTRASOUND WILL EITHER BACK THIS UP OR GIVE A MORE ACCURATE ESTIMATED DUE DATE.

ULTRASOUND: WITH A WAND THAT GOES INTO YOUR VAGINA. SOME DOCTORS WILL OFFER FOR YOU TO STICK IT INSIDE YOURSELF, WHICH IS PRETTY COOL.

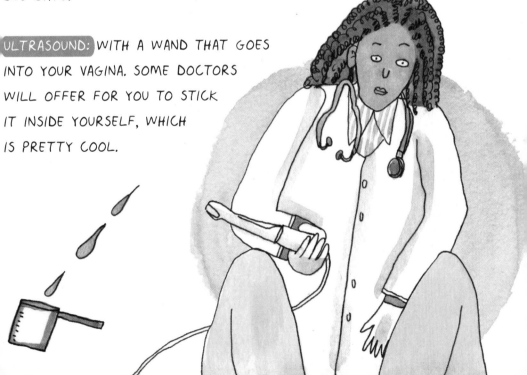

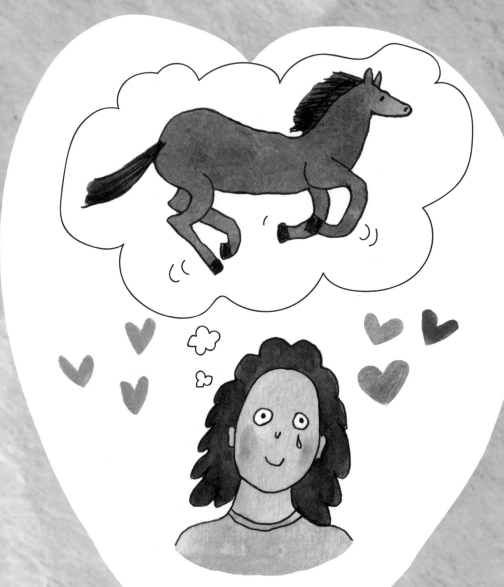

DURING THE ULTRASOUND YOU'LL HEAR THE BABY'S HEARTBEAT FOR THE FIRST TIME. THE HEARTBEAT SOUNDS LIKE GALLOPING HORSES. IT CAN BE AN EMOTIONAL AND BEAUTIFUL MOMENT.

Not Alone

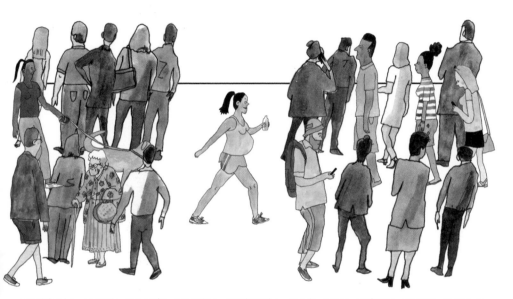

HEARING YOUR BABY'S HEART BEATING FOR THE FIRST TIME WHILE INSIDE YOU IS A TREMENDOUS EXPERIENCE. POSSIBLY ONE THAT'S HARD TO IMAGINE IF YOU HAVEN'T BEEN THERE. MOMENTS LIKE THIS AND ALL THE BIG CHANGES THAT COME ALONG WITH PREGNANCY ARE WHY IT'S IMPORTANT TO HAVE A SUPPORT GROUP WHILE YOU'RE PREGNANT. IN THE MOMENT, BEING PREGNANT IS THE BIGGEST DEAL, BUT THEN YOU HAVE A NEWBORN, AND YOU HAVE TO QUICKLY MOVE ON. THERE'S NOT REALLY ENOUGH TIME TO PROCESS YOUR EXPERIENCE AFTER THE BABY IS BORN. FINDING A COMMUNITY WHILE PREGNANT IS A NECESSARY STEP IN GETTING THE MOST OUT OF THE EXPERIENCE. WHAT FOLLOWS ARE SOME IDEAS ON HOW TO DO THIS.

FIND A BUDDY

MANY PEOPLE WILL POST ABOUT THEIR PREGNANCIES ON SOCIAL MEDIA, AND IT'S LIKELY THAT AN OLD FRIEND OR COWORKER WILL BE PREGNANT AT THE SAME TIME AS YOU. FEEL FREE TO REACH OUT TO THEM AND ASK TO HANG. YOU'RE BOTH GOING TO EXPERIENCE A LOT OF CHANGES AND SPECIAL MOMENTS, AND IT'S INVALUABLE TO HAVE SOMEONE TO TEXT/CALL/HANG WITH WHO UNDERSTANDS PRETTY MUCH EXACTLY HOW YOU FEEL. BONUS POINTS IF YOUR DUE DATES ARE CLOSE TOGETHER.

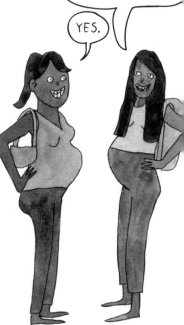

LET'S GO FIND THE BATHROOM.

YES.

REDDIT SUBS

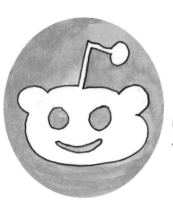

GOOGLE IS GENERALLY A GREAT SOURCE FOR INFORMATION, BUT WHEN YOU'RE PREGNANT THERE IS LOTS OF WORST–CASE–SCENARIO STUFF ON THERE—MAYBE STUFF YOU'D RATHER NOT FOCUS ON. HOWEVER, REDDIT GROUPS LIKE "R/PREGNANT" AND "R/BABYBUMPS" ARE GREAT FOR ASKING QUESTIONS AND READING ABOUT OTHERS' EXPERIENCES. LESS SPOOKINESS, MORE COMMUNITY.

PERHAPS YOUR GRANDMA DIDN'T GET NAUSEOUS (LIKE YOU!), MAYBE YOUR COWORKER HAD TO BE INDUCED FOR ALL THREE OF HER BIRTHS, MAYBE YOUR MENTOR HAD A C-SECTION AFTER LABORING FOR A FEW DAYS. HEARING FIRSTHAND STORIES FROM PEOPLE YOU KNOW WILL HELP YOU FEEL LESS ALONE AND MORE CONNECTED DURING THIS TIME OF CHANGE.

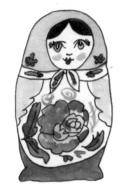
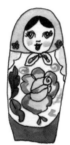
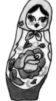

READ BIRTH STORIES

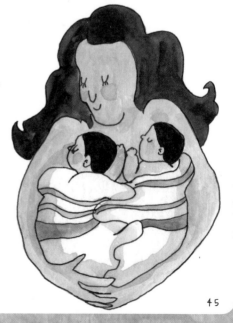

MAYBE YOU'RE HAVING TWINS AND YOU DON'T PERSONALLY KNOW ANYONE WHO HAD TWINS. OR MAYBE YOU WANT A WATERBIRTH, BUT YOU DON'T KNOW ANYONE WHO HAD ONE. IF YOU CAN, FIND STORIES ON SPECIFICALLY WHAT YOU WANT AND READ THEM TO HELP YOU IMAGINE WHAT YOUR BABY'S BIRTH WILL BE LIKE.

45

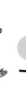

GETTING THE ANSWERS

DURING THE GENETIC SCREENING YOU HAD THE OPTION TO FIND OUT THE SEX. THE DOCTOR TOLD YOU THEY WOULD LEAVE A VOICEMAIL AND AT THE END SAY "BOY" OR "GIRL" AND THAT YOU COULD WAIT TO HEAR IT WITH YOUR PARTNER. THAT SOUNDED LIKE A GREAT IDEA SO YOU WAITED ALL DAY TO HEAR IT WITH HIM. YOU WERE REALLY, REALLY NERVOUS AND EXCITED TO HEAR AND IT WAS A HUGE BUILDUP. FINALLY THE VOICEMAIL GOT TO THE END AND IT SAID:

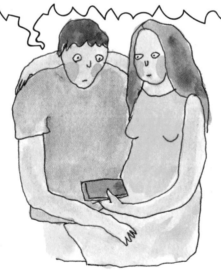

LOOKS LIKE YOU REQUESTED TO KNOW THE GENDER, BUT IT WAS HARD TO DETERMINE SO WE'LL CALL YOU BACK NEXT WEEK TO LET YOU KNOW.

SO ANTICLIMACTIC!

YOU'VE GOT IT IN YOU

IT STARTS POURING OUT OF NOWHERE WHILE YOU ARE RIDING YOUR BIKE. AT FIRST, YOU ARE A LITTLE AFRAID, SINCE IT'S SLIPPERY AND YOUR BRAKES HARDLY WORK IN THE RAIN. HOWEVER, YOU ARE PREPARED WITH A PONCHO AND AS YOU RIDE, YOU ARE OVERCOME BY A FEELING THAT YOU KNOW YOU CAN TAKE CARE OF YOUR BABY. A FEELING THAT YOU WILL BE OK, THAT THIS MOMENT IS JUST PART OF A GREAT ADVENTURE YOU ARE STARTING TOGETHER.

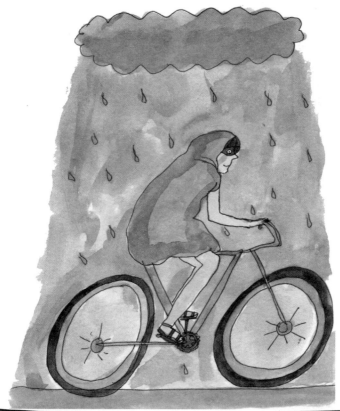

I'M NOT DRINKING RIGHT NOW...

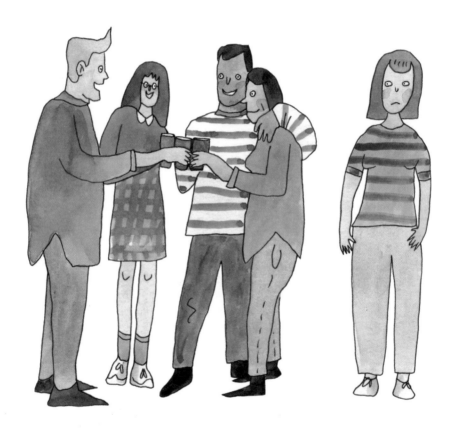

YOU GO TO A SAINT PATRICK'S DAY BRUNCH WHERE EVERYONE AND THEIR MOM IS DRINKING. YOU ARE A BIT OF A PARTY ANIMAL, SO SOBRIETY IS A STRANGE LOOK ON YOU.

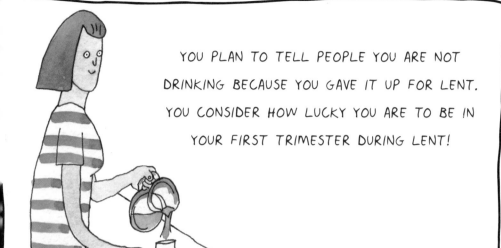

YOU PLAN TO TELL PEOPLE YOU ARE NOT DRINKING BECAUSE YOU GAVE IT UP FOR LENT. YOU CONSIDER HOW LUCKY YOU ARE TO BE IN YOUR FIRST TRIMESTER DURING LENT!

YOU SEE A FRIEND AND WALK OVER TO HIM. HE'S MAKING BLOODY MARYS.

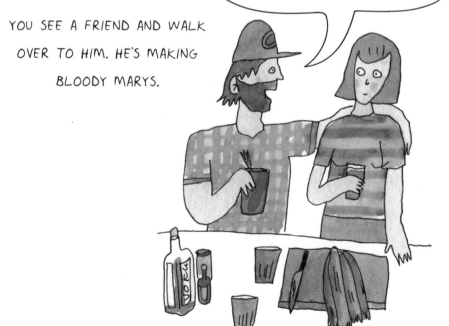

WOULD YOU LIKE ONE?

YOU TRY TO SAY THAT YOU ARE DRINKING A VIRGIN DRINK BUT INSTEAD MUMBLE...

OH NO...UM I'M HAVING A LITTLE BABY, I MEAN, A VIRGIN, YOU KNOW—"BABY DRINK."

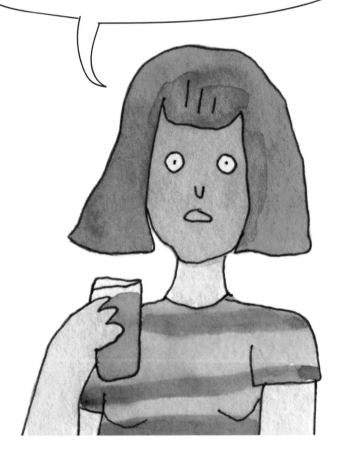

HE LOOKS AT YOU INCREDULOUSLY.

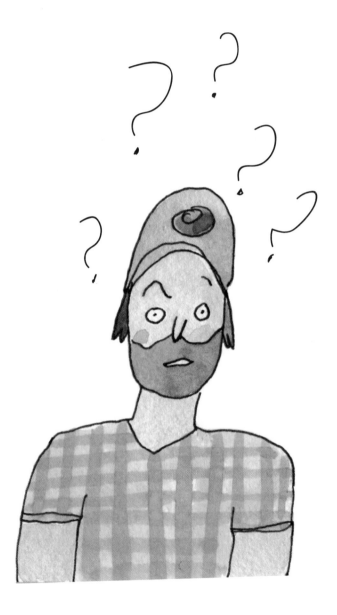

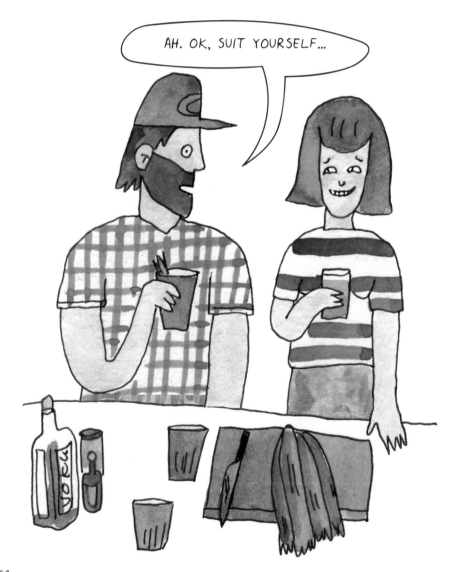

At Three Months

TINY SKINNY HUMAN

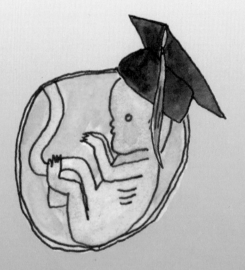

WEEKS
9-13

CONGRATS, YOUR BABY HAS GRADUATED FROM AN EMBRYO
TO A FETUS AND NO LONGER HAS A TAIL.

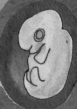

AVERAGE END-OF-MONTH SIZE: 2.91 IN (7.4 CM)

DRESS SHOPPING

YOU'RE INVITED TO A WEDDING AT WHICH POINT YOU'LL BE FIVE MONTHS PREGNANT. SO FAR IT'S NOT OBVIOUS THAT YOU'RE PREGNANT AT ALL, EVEN THOUGH YOUR PANTS FEEL A LITTLE TIGHT. YOU DON'T KNOW WHAT YOU'LL LOOK LIKE IN A COUPLE MONTHS SO YOU DECIDE TO GOOGLE WHAT A FIVE-MONTH BELLY LOOKS LIKE AS YOU ARE ONLINE SHOPPING FOR YOUR DRESS.

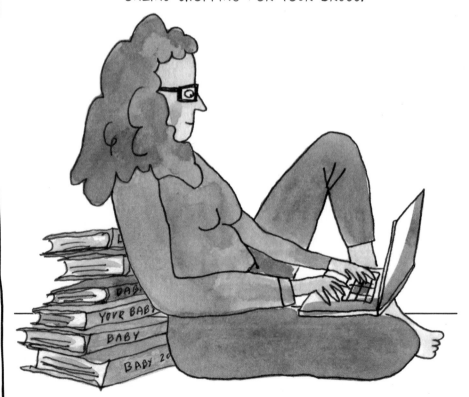

YOU SEE ALL TYPES OF BODY SHAPES—TYPICAL. NOTHING IN PREGNANCY IS ONE SIZE FITS ALL. AS YOU KEEP SCROLLING, YOU SEE SOMEONE WHO'S FOUR MONTHS PREGNANT WITH A SIX-PACK.

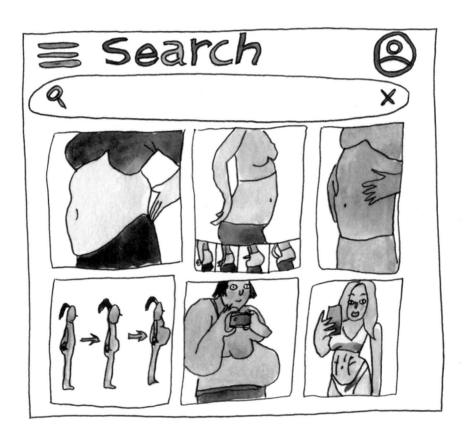

AT FIRST YOU'RE LIKE:

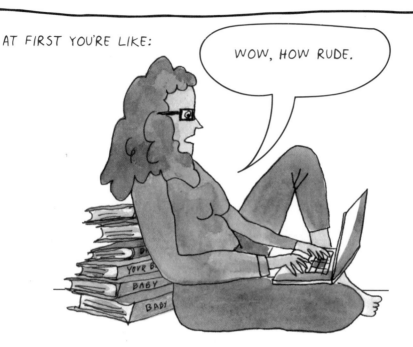

WOW, HOW RUDE.

BUT THEN YOU LAUGH AS YOU REALIZE THE ABSURDITY OF THE

SITUATION AND GOOGLE FIND.

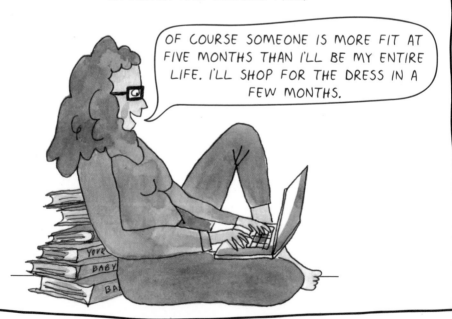

OF COURSE SOMEONE IS MORE FIT AT FIVE MONTHS THAN I'LL BE MY ENTIRE LIFE. I'LL SHOP FOR THE DRESS IN A FEW MONTHS.

A LOT MORE BODILY FLUIDS...

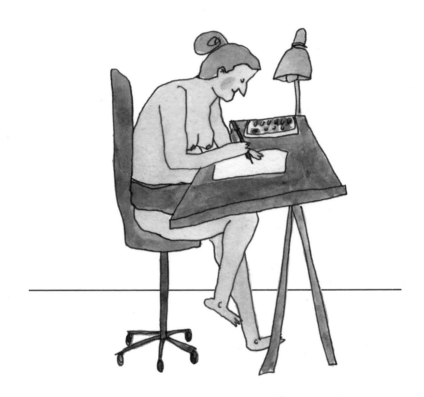

ONE HOT SUMMER DAY YOU ARE NATURALLY DRAWING IN YOUR UNDERWEAR (WHY PAY MORE FOR AIR-CONDITIONING?) AND YOU LOOK DOWN TO SEE LIQUID COMING OUT OF YOUR NIPPLES! IT IS BOTH AMAZING AND GROSS AT THE SAME TIME. YOU FEEL SOME PEACE OF MIND, SINCE YOU CAN SEE THAT YOUR BODY IS GETTING READY!

NORMALIZE LOSS

ABOUT ONE IN FOUR PREGNANCIES ENDS IN MISCARRIAGE. EVEN THOUGH IT'S SO COMMON, IT CAN BE DEVASTATING. IT'S FRUSTRATING: WE'RE NOT SUPPOSED TO TELL PEOPLE WE'RE PREGNANT IN THE FIRST TRIMESTER BECAUSE THIS MIGHT HAPPEN, BUT THEN WHEN IT HAPPENS, WHO IS THERE TO SUPPORT US WITH OUR LOSS?

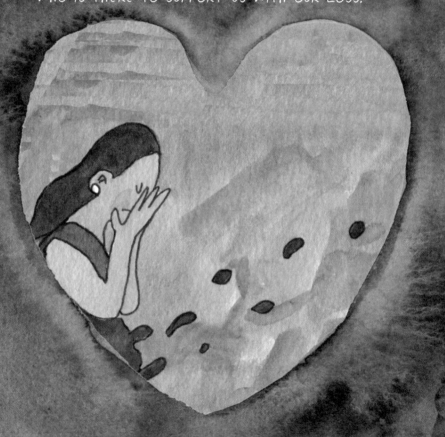

PERHAPS IT'S TIME WE START TALKING ABOUT IT MORE, AND WHILE WE'RE AT IT, CAN WE COME UP WITH A BETTER NAME? MISCARRIAGE SOUNDS LIKE SOMEONE FELL OUT OF THEIR VICTORIAN-ERA VEHICLE.

MIZUKO KUYŌ

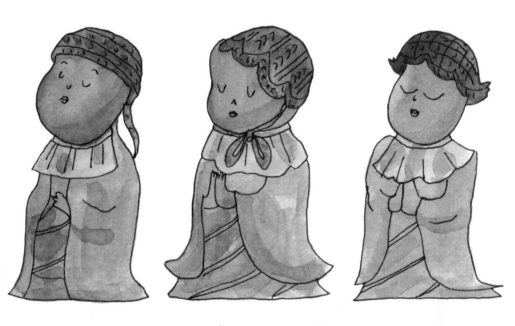

IN FACT, IN JAPAN, THEY HAVE "MIZUKO KUYŌ," WHICH TRANSLATES TO "WATER CHILD MEMORIAL SERVICE." IT IS A CEREMONY THAT A PARENT PRACTICES WHEN THEY EXPERIENCE A STILLBIRTH, MISCARRIAGE, OR ABORTION. WHILE IT IS NOT FREE FROM ITS OWN CONTROVERSIES, IT WOULD BE NICE TO HAVE SOMETHING LIKE THIS IN PLACE ALL OVER THE WORLD TO HELP PEOPLE DEAL WITH THE FEELINGS THAT COME UP DURING A LOSS.

First Trimester

BY THE END OF THE FIRST TRIMESTER YOU WILL LIKELY HAVE
ACCOMPLISHED THE FOLLOWING:

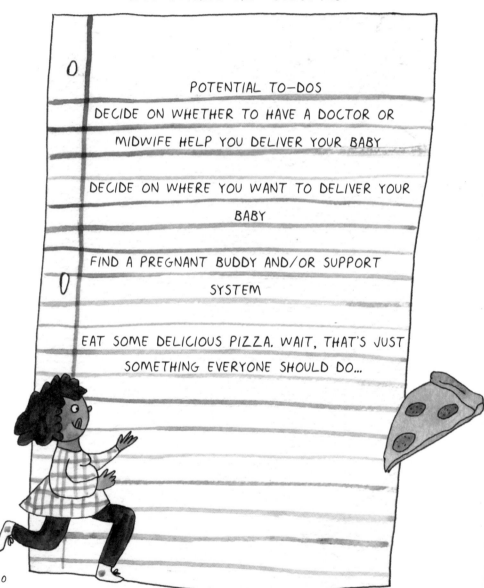

POTENTIAL TO-DOS

DECIDE ON WHETHER TO HAVE A DOCTOR OR
MIDWIFE HELP YOU DELIVER YOUR BABY

DECIDE ON WHERE YOU WANT TO DELIVER YOUR
BABY

FIND A PREGNANT BUDDY AND/OR SUPPORT
SYSTEM

EAT SOME DELICIOUS PIZZA. WAIT, THAT'S JUST
SOMETHING EVERYONE SHOULD DO...

Second Trimester

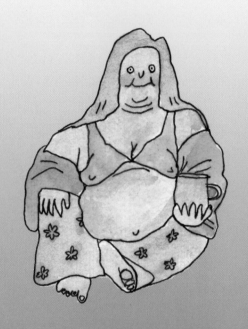

BEST TRIMESTER(?)

Second-Trimester Feelings

FEELING BIGGER AND, HOPEFULLY, BETTER

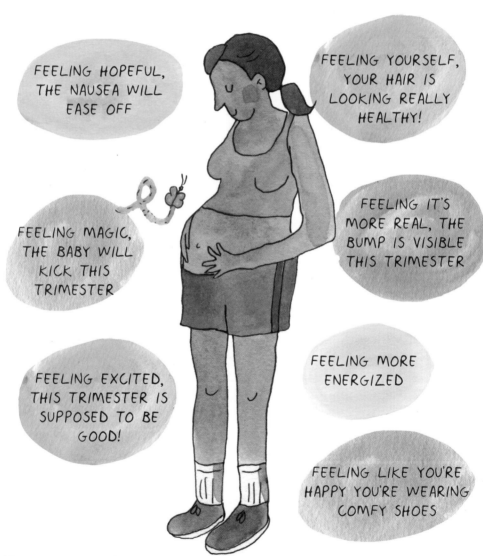

At Four Months

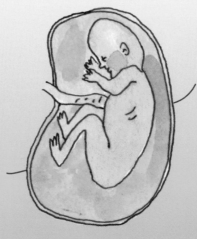

CAN HEAR
SOUNDS

VISIBLE
GENITALS

WEEKS
14–17

FOUR MONTHS CAN FEEL LIKE A TRANSITION PERIOD. NO
LONGER IN YOUR FIRST TRIMESTER, BUT MAYBE NOT FULLY IN
THE SWING OF THE SECOND TRIMESTER EITHER.

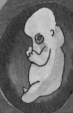

AVERAGE END-OF-MONTH SIZE: 4.57 IN (11.6 CM)

The Nursery

THE SECOND TRIMESTER CAN BE A GREAT TIME TO START GETTING THE NURSERY TOGETHER. THIS CAN BE A FUN PART OF BEING PREGNANT! THERE ARE SO MANY WAYS TO CREATE A NURSERY AND SO MANY TYPES OF NURSERIES. BONUS—CREATIVE PROJECTS LIKE THIS ONE CAN HELP A PERSON PROCESS CHANGE AND GROWTH.

BLACKOUT CURTAINS: WON'T NEED THESE AT FIRST, BUT CAN BE HELPFUL A FEW MONTHS IN.

BABY MONITOR: CAMERA OR SOUND? OR NONE AT ALL?

CHANGING AREA: DOESN'T HAVE TO BE LOCATED IN THE NURSERY, BUT DEFINITELY NICE TO HAVE ONE CLOSE BY. CAN USE YOUR OWN BED.

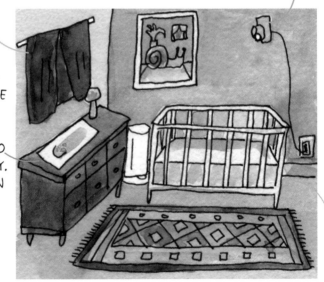

PLACE FOR BABY TO SLEEP: THIS IS THE ONLY THING YOU REALLY NEED, AND EVEN THEN, YOU MIGHT HAVE A BASSINET OR COSLEEPER BY YOUR BED AT FIRST.

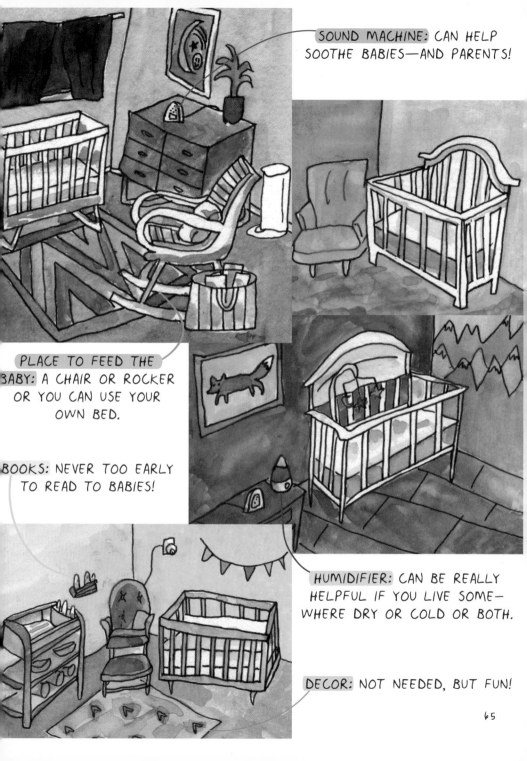

SOUND MACHINE: CAN HELP SOOTHE BABIES—AND PARENTS!

PLACE TO FEED THE BABY: A CHAIR OR ROCKER OR YOU CAN USE YOUR OWN BED.

BOOKS: NEVER TOO EARLY TO READ TO BABIES!

HUMIDIFIER: CAN BE REALLY HELPFUL IF YOU LIVE SOME—WHERE DRY OR COLD OR BOTH.

DECOR: NOT NEEDED, BUT FUN!

"IT WAS MY FAVORITE TRIMESTER"

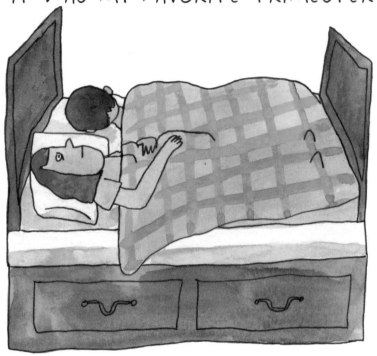

PEOPLE TOLD YOU IT WAS SUPPOSED TO GET EASIER IN THE SECOND TRIMESTER. BUT YOU'RE NOT BUYING IT. YOU'RE HAVING SUCH A HARD TIME SLEEPING THAT YOU HAD TO DEVELOP A SLEEP PLAN. NOW THAT YOU'VE DRASTICALLY VEERED FROM "THE NORM," YOU'VE HAD TO CONFRONT THE FACT THAT THERE IS NO NORM, AND YOU'VE RESOLVED TO THINK OF THE BENCHMARKS AS POTENTIAL OUTCOMES, NOT RULES TO HOLD ON TO.

EVERY PREGNANCY IS DIFFERENT: YOU WEREN'T VERY SICK THE FIRST TRIMESTER, BUT THE SECOND ONE STARTED OFF REALLY ROUGH.

SLEEP PLAN DETAILS

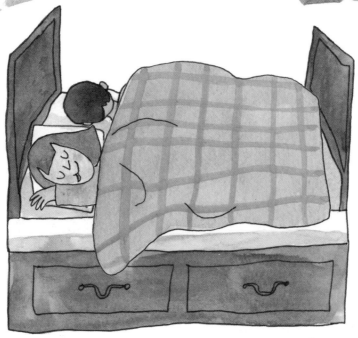

RULES

- IN BED BY 9:15 PM
- NO PHONE IN BED UNLESS PODCAST
- READ IN BED (NO PHONE!)
- STAY IN BED UNTIL 7:15 AM EVEN IF I WAKE UP EARLIER

TOOLS

- CALM MY THOUGHTS THROUGH BREATHS
- IF WORRIED, CREATE A TO-DO LIST AT 8 PM
- USE PHYSICAL COMFORT: TENSE AND RELAX MUSCLES
- NO/LITTLE LIGHT IN BEDROOM
- EAT SOMETHING IF I CAN'T SLEEP

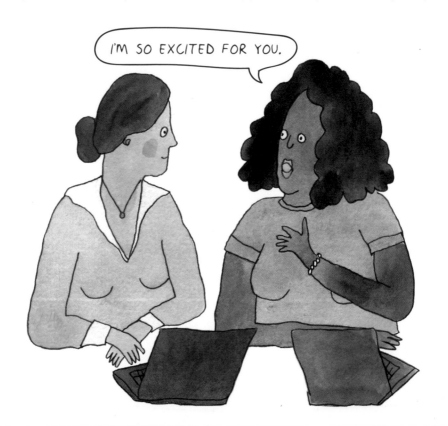

TELLING YOUR BOSS

ONCE THE SECOND TRIMESTER IS REACHED, MOST PEOPLE LET THE CAT OUT OF THE BAG AT THE WORKPLACE. EVEN THOUGH IT SHOULDN'T BE, TELLING YOUR BOSS CAN BE STRESSFUL, AWKWARD, AND SOME- TIMES EVEN SCARY. IT'S HELPFUL TO HAVE A PLAN OF HOW AND WHEN YOU'LL TELL THEM. THEY MAY BE DISAPPOINTED OR STRESSED BY THE NEWS FOR BUSINESS-RELATED REASONS, BUT THE ONLY APPROPRIATE REACTION FROM THEM IS TO BE SUPPORTIVE AND CONGRATULATORY.

BABY GROWS ON YOU

AS TIME GOES ON, YOU START TO GIVE THE BABY MORE AND MORE OF A PERSONALITY. SOMETIMES, FOR FUN, YOU PRETEND TO BE THE BABY TALKING TO YOUR PARTNER. YOU TALK TO HIM IN THE VOICE OF "TONY" FROM "THE SHINING." STILL MAKES YOU LAUGH TO THINK ABOUT IT. YOUR PARTNER, NOT SO MUCH.

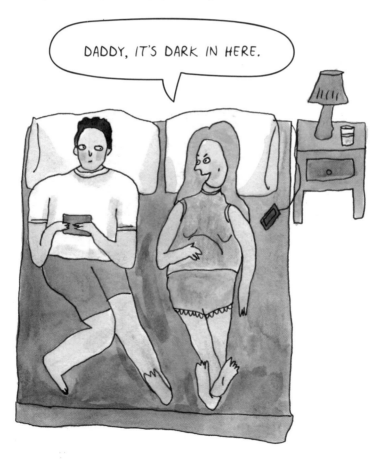

DADDY, IT'S DARK IN HERE.

Eating

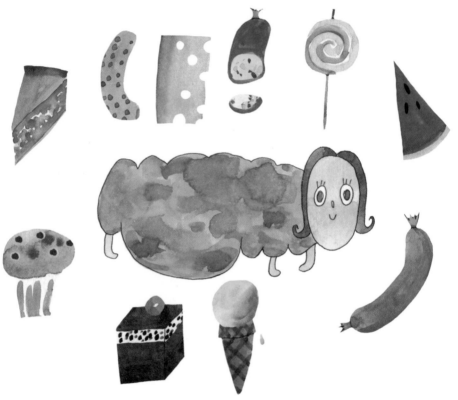

TO BE PREGNANT AND FREE OF NAUSEA IS TO EXPERIENCE THE INSATIABLE URGE TO EAT. THERE'S A LOT OF HYPE ABOUT HOW PREGNANT WOMEN CAN'T EAT CERTAIN FOODS. WHAT ISN'T MENTIONED IS ALL THE THINGS A PREGNANT WOMAN CAN (AND SHOULD) EAT. ALMOST ALL THE FOOD! WHY IS THE EMPHASIS SO NEGATIVE? IT'S TIME TO RECLAIM AND RELISH THIS HUNGRY TIME. ABOUT 300—500 EXTRA CALORIES PER DAY ARE NEEDED IN THE SECOND AND THIRD TRIMESTERS. THAT'S ABOUT 2 DONUTS PER DAY, IF YOU WANT TO MEASURE IN DONUTS.

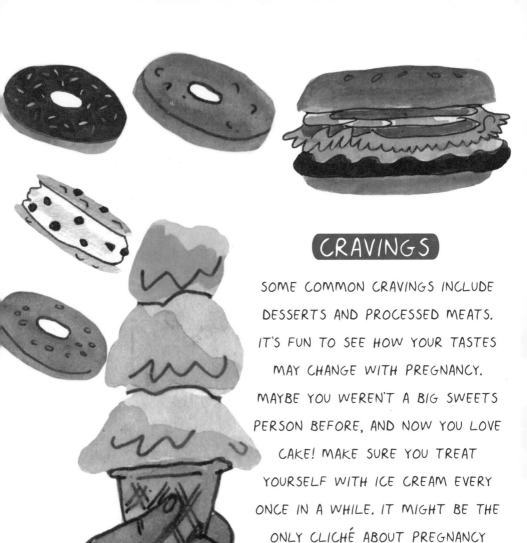

CRAVINGS

SOME COMMON CRAVINGS INCLUDE
DESSERTS AND PROCESSED MEATS.
IT'S FUN TO SEE HOW YOUR TASTES
MAY CHANGE WITH PREGNANCY.
MAYBE YOU WEREN'T A BIG SWEETS
PERSON BEFORE, AND NOW YOU LOVE
CAKE! MAKE SURE YOU TREAT
YOURSELF WITH ICE CREAM EVERY
ONCE IN A WHILE. IT MIGHT BE THE
ONLY CLICHÉ ABOUT PREGNANCY
THAT IS TRULY UNIVERSAL.

BUT BE CAUTIOUS...

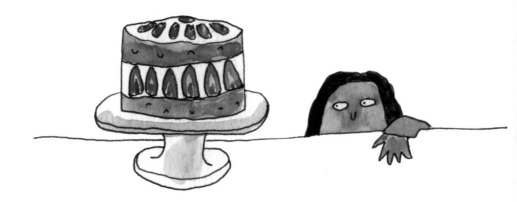

IF THERE'S AN ENTIRE CAKE IN FRONT OF ANYONE WHO'S LITERALLY GROWING A BABY, IT MAY BE DIFFICULT TO STOP.

OR NOT... DO WHATEVER YOU WANT.

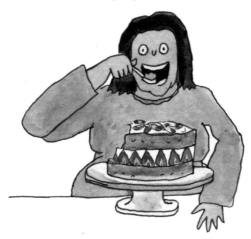

At Five Months

DUDE LOOKS LIKE A BABY!

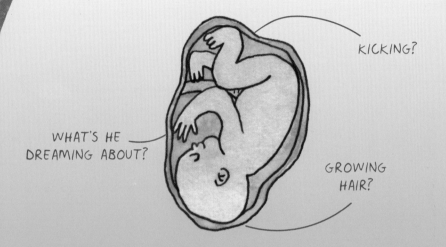

KICKING?

WHAT'S HE
DREAMING ABOUT?

GROWING
HAIR?

WEEKS
18-22

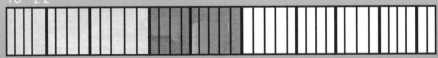

YOU'RE HALFWAY THERE! MOST WOMEN WILL BE
SHOWING BY NOW AND HOPEFULLY BENEFITING FROM
MORE ENERGY AND LESS NAUSEA!

AVERAGE END-OF-MONTH SIZE: 10.51 IN (26.7 CM)

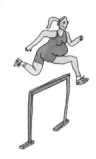

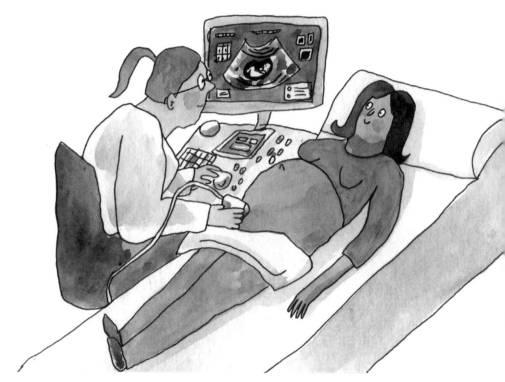

THE 20-WEEK ULTRASOUND
HAPPENS BETWEEN 18 AND 21 WEEKS

DURING THIS EXCITING APPOINTMENT THE TALENTED ULTRASOUND TECH WILL ZOOM IN AND EXAMINE ALL THE TINY, TINY BABY PARTS. THIS CAN TAKE A LONG TIME IF THE BABY ISN'T COOPERATING, BUT YOU MIGHT NOT CARE, BECAUSE YOU'LL BE SEEING YOUR BABY IN GREAT DETAIL! AFTERWARDS, THEY'LL PRINT YOU OUT SOME PHOTOS FOR THE FRIDGE.

74

DO IT YOUR WAY

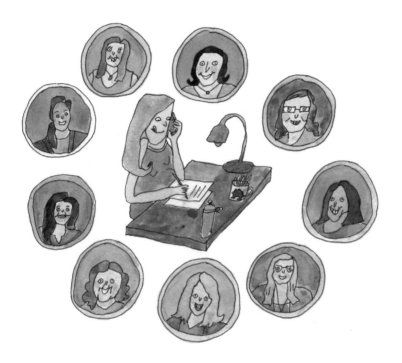

AFTER READING THAT YOU ARE 28% LESS LIKELY TO HAVE A C-SECTION WITH A DOULA, YOU DECIDE YOU WILL GET ONE. YOU INTERVIEW NINE DOULAS TO FIND THE RIGHT ONE. EACH TIME YOU TALK WITH ONE, YOU LEARN SOMETHING NEW ABOUT LABOR AND BIRTHING A HUMAN.

YOU END UP GOING WITH ONE WHO YOU REALLY VIBE WITH. SHE HAS A CALMING PRESENCE AND FITS YOUR PRICE RANGE.

YOU ADMIT YOU WENT OVERBOARD WITH THE INTERVIEWS. BUT YOU DON'T REGRET IT, YOU LEARNED A LOT. THE DOULAS DROPPED SOME KNOWLEDGE ON YOU, INCLUDING:

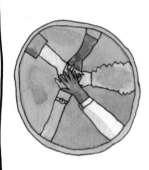

EVERYONE HAS PRIORITIES: YOU HAVE A BIRTH TEAM AND EACH PERSON ON THE TEAM HAS A ROLE AND GOAL. FOR EXAMPLE, YOUR DOCTOR/MIDWIFE IS THINKING ABOUT ANY POTENTIAL MEDICAL RISKS. BEING ABLE TO SEE THINGS FROM THEIR PERSPECTIVE MIGHT GIVE YOU INSIGHT ON WHY THEY MAY DO OR SAY SOMETHING.

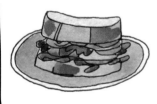

EAT BEFORE YOU GO: AS LONG AS YOUR DOCTOR DIDN'T SPECIFICALLY TELL YOU NOT TO, YOU SHOULD EAT BEFORE YOU GO TO THE HOSPITAL BECAUSE ONCE YOU ARE THERE, THEY MAY KEEP YOU ON AN ALL—LIQUID DIET. IF YOU'RE ABLE, BRING YOUR FAVORITE SNACKS AND SPORTS DRINKS TO GIVE YOU ENERGY DURING LABOR.

EPIDURALS WEAR OFF: YOU WERE SORT OF WORRIED ABOUT GETTING AN EPIDURAL, SO YOU ASKED YOUR DOULA INTERVIEWEES ABOUT THIS A LOT. EVEN THOUGH THE EXPERIENCE CAN VARY, YOU LEARN THAT GENERALLY YOU GET A SHOT THAT MAKES YOU NUMB, THEN YOU GET A LITTLE REMOTE—CONTROL THING THAT YOU PUSH IF YOU WANT MORE.

ADDITIONALLY, YOU LEARN THAT IF YOU GET AN EPIDURAL, EVERYONE HAS TO LEAVE THE ROOM EXCEPT FOR THE PREGNANT WOMAN AND THE HOSPITAL STAFF. "SOMETHING TO DO WITH HUSBANDS FAINTING IN THE PAST," A DOULA HALF—JOKES WHEN YOU ASK WHY.*

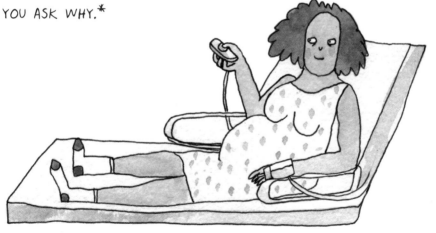

*THEY'RE MINIMIZING RISKS LIKE CONTAMINATION WHEN ASKING NONMEDICAL PEOPLE TO LEAVE.

BUY for BABY

GETTING STUFF FOR YOUR NEW FAMILY MEMBER IS FUN, STRESSFUL, AND INEVITABLE. THERE ARE FAR TOO MANY PRODUCTS OUT THERE FOR NEW BABIES, BUT ONE THING YOU'LL DEFINITELY NEED IS A PLACE TO STORE YOUR BABY ONCE IT'S NO LONGER INSIDE YOU.

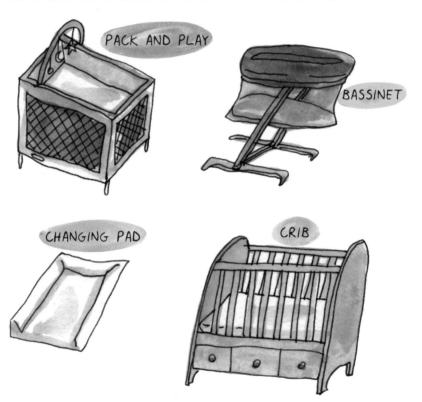

PACK AND PLAY

BASSINET

CHANGING PAD

CRIB

YOU PURCHASE ALL THE ITEMS THAT YOU THINK ARE ESSENTIAL BUT CAN'T POSSIBLY BE, AND YOU FINALLY THINK YOU'RE ALL SET...

...WHEN YOU REALIZE YOU ALSO HAVE TO BUY FITTED SHEETS FOR ALL OF THOSE BABY CONTAINERS! AND THEY HAVE TO FIT EXACTLY OR ELSE IT'S SUPER DANGEROUS?? IT FEELS LIKE THE BUYING NEVER ENDS, AND AFTER A WHILE YOU DECIDE YOU JUST HAVE ENOUGH STUFF (MAYBE).

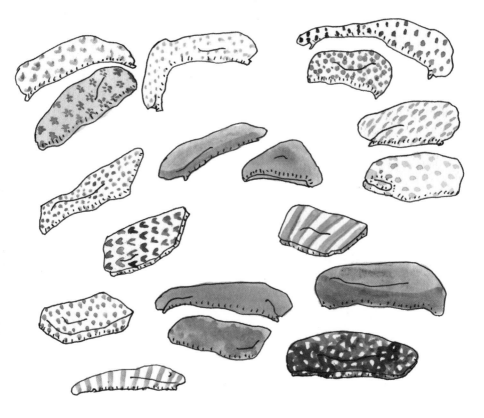

ON YOUR QUEST TO PROVIDE FOR YOUR CHILD, YOU GO DOWN A BUNCH OF RABBIT HOLES FOR DIFFERENT ITEMS. YOU WOULD HAVE NEVER GUESSED THERE WERE THAT MANY TYPES OF STROLLERS, CRIBS, OR CHANGING PADS—OR THAT YOU COULD LEARN SO MUCH ABOUT EACH.

CHANGING PADS!

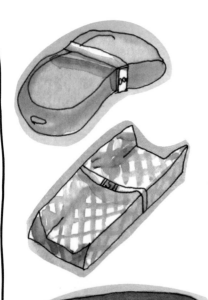

$130
★★★★★

MOTTO: "YOU WANT THE BEST FOR YOUR KID, DON'T YOU?"
TWIST: COSTS $5 MORE FOR A GENDER-NEUTRAL COLOR.

$25
★★★★⯨

MOTTO: "OK, I GUESS, FOR SOME BABIES."
TWIST: IT'S SERIOUSLY OK FOR ANY BABY.

$150
★★★★★

MOTTO: "THIS ONE PAIRS WITH YOUR PHONE, 'CAUSE WHY NOT?"
TWIST: THERE IS ABSOLUTELY NO REASON TO PAIR A CHANGING PAD TO YOUR PHONE.

$18
★★★★⯨

MOTTO: "NONE OF THESE PRODUCTS CAN GET LESS THAN FOUR AND A HALF STARS."
TWIST: THEY LITERALLY ALL WORK FINE. A TOWEL WOULD WORK.

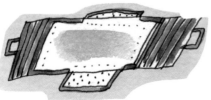

IT'S OVERWHELMING, EXCITING, AND TIRING. ONE THING IS FOR SURE: THE BEST ITEMS ARE THE HAND-ME-DOWNS. WHILE SOME USED BABY PRODUCTS NO LONGER MEET SAFETY STANDARDS, THE ONES THAT CAN BE REPURPOSED ARE THE BEST. THEY'RE TRIED, PROVEN, AND FREE!

At Six Months

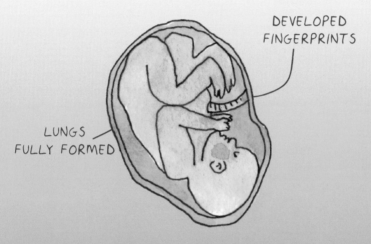

DEVELOPED
FINGERPRINTS

LUNGS
FULLY FORMED

WEEKS
23–27

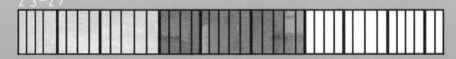

THIS IS A BIG MONTH FOR BABY. ACCORDING TO SOME STUDIES, BABIES GO FROM 20–35% SURVIVAL IF BORN PREMATURELY AT 24 WEEKS TO 50–70% AT 25 WEEKS, AND MORE THAN 90% AT 26 TO 27 WEEKS.

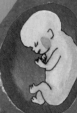

AVERAGE END-OF-MONTH SIZE: 14.41 IN (36.6 CM)

Preemie

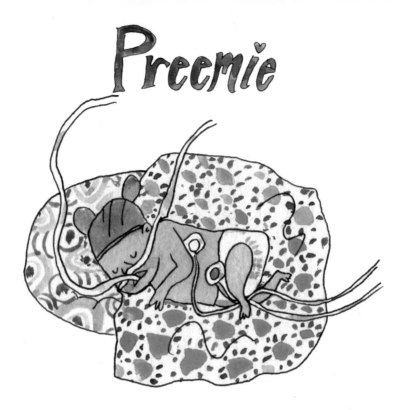

SPEAKING OF BEING BORN PREMATURELY, IN THE USA, ABOUT ONE IN TEN
BABIES ARE BORN PRETERM, OR BEFORE 37 WEEKS. IN MOST CASES
PRETERM LABOR STARTS UNEXPECTEDLY AND THE REASON IS UNKNOWN.

HOSPITALS HAVE LEVELS OF NICU SUPPORT, WITH THE HIGHEST BEING A
LEVEL 4 NICU, CAPABLE OF CARING FOR BABIES AS YOUNG AS 22 WEEKS.

THERE'S NOTHING MORE HEARTBREAKING THAN HAVING TO LEAVE YOUR BABY
AT THE HOSPITAL. THERE ARE SUPPORT GROUPS OUT THERE TO HELP
PARENTS IN THIS SITUATION.

SLEEPING TROUBLES

PREGNANCY HAS MADE SLEEP DIFFICULT, BUT BY SIX MONTHS IT'S AT A WHOLE NEW LEVEL. FORTUNATELY, YOU HAVE ADAPTED WITH AN ENTIRE PILLOW SYSTEM, AND YOU RECENTLY MOVED TO A BIGGER, COOLER BEDROOM. ONE NIGHT, YOU GO TO BED AT 8 PM BECAUSE YOU LITERALLY CAN'T HOLD YOURSELF IN A SEATED POSITION ANY LONGER. YOU WAKE UP AROUND ONE AM WITH YOUR BACK HURTING, BUT CONTINUE TO TRY TO SLEEP INTERMITTENTLY FOR A COUPLE HOURS.

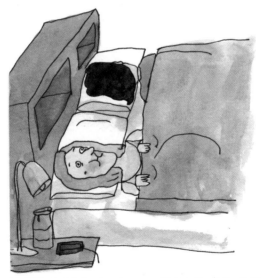

BY 4 AM, YOU CAN'T SLEEP, SO YOU GET UP AND HAVE SOME CEREAL AND TAKE A WARM SHOWER. YOU ALSO GET A HEATING PAD FOR YOUR BACK. YOU ARE ABLE TO FALL ASLEEP AFTER THAT, ONLY TO WAKE YOURSELF UP A COUPLE HOURS LATER BY PUKING IN YOUR MOUTH. ONE OF THOSE "SO TERRIBLE IT'S FUNNY" MOMENTS.

FOOD IS A BIG DEAL!

YOU ARE HAVING PRETTY BAD HEARTBURN AND FOR THREE WEEKS YOU TRY TO IGNORE IT. FINALLY ONE NIGHT IT IS SO BAD YOUR PARTNER OFFERS TO GO GET ANTACIDS. WHEN HE IS LEAVING, HE ASKS IF YOU NEED OR WANT ANYTHING ELSE. YOU SAY CAKE.

WHILE HE IS GONE YOU ALMOST PUKE FROM THE HEARTBURN. WHEN HE RETURNS HE HAS BOUGHT YOU THREE DIFFERENT KINDS OF CAKE. YOU ARE SO HAPPY THAT YOU CRY.

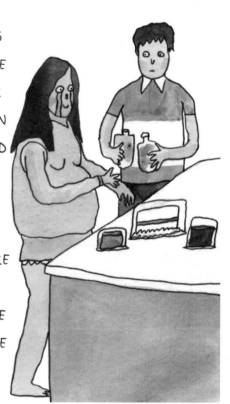

HEARTBURN CURES

CURE	DIFFICULTY LEVEL
AVOID FOODS THAT MAKE YOU FEEL SICK (DUH!)	MEDIUM: IF YOU CAN PINPOINT SOMETHING THAT MAKES YOU SICK AND AVOID IT, THAT'S A WIN. IF YOU PINPOINT SOMETHING THAT MAKES YOU SICK AND YOU CRAVE IT FOR A WEEK STRAIGHT, THAT'S A BIT HARDER.
EAT SMALLER MEALS THROUGHOUT THE DAY	EASY(?): YOU ARE HUNGRY ALL THE TIME, SO EATING FREQUENTLY IS A MUST. EATING SMALLER MEALS IS EASY IN THEORY (SINCE YOU LITERALLY DON'T HAVE SPACE FOR BIG MEALS) BUT IT'S DIFFICULT TO DETERMINE HOW SMALL A SMALL MEAL ACTUALLY NEEDS TO BE...
ANTACIDS	MEDIUM: IT'S EASY TO TAKE THEM, IT'S DIFFICULT TO STOP.
DON'T EAT TOO CLOSE TO GOING TO BED OR LYING DOWN	EXTREMELY DIFFICULT: ALL YOU WANT TO DO IS EAT AND REST, SO THIS ADVICE IS PRETTY MUCH GARBAGE AT THIS POINT.

TALK TO YOUR DOCTOR IF THE ABOVE DOESN'T HELP.

THE PREGNANCY CONUNDRUM

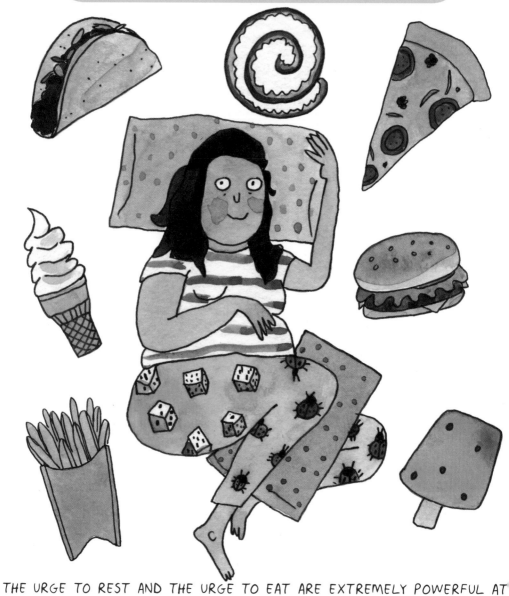

THE URGE TO REST AND THE URGE TO EAT ARE EXTREMELY POWERFUL AT THIS POINT. YOU WANT SO BADLY TO JUST LIE ABOUT, BUT WHEN YOU LIE DOWN, YOU THINK OF ALL THE NICE DELICIOUS FOOD YOU COULD BE EATING

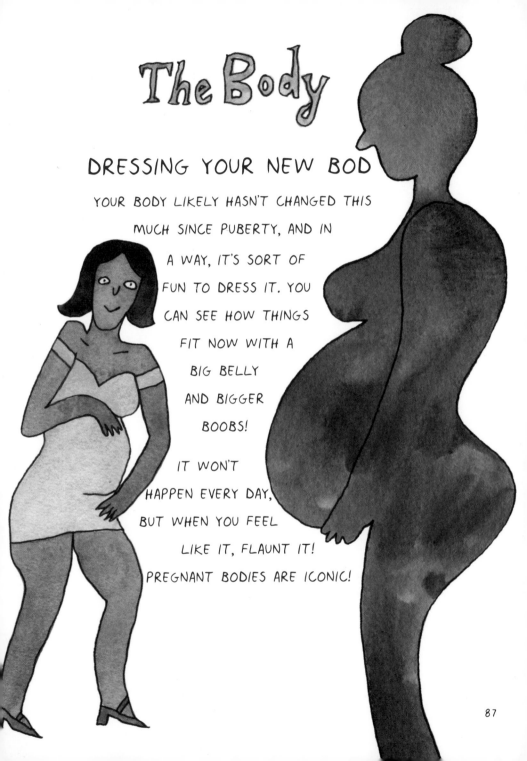

The Body

DRESSING YOUR NEW BOD

YOUR BODY LIKELY HASN'T CHANGED THIS MUCH SINCE PUBERTY, AND IN A WAY, IT'S SORT OF FUN TO DRESS IT. YOU CAN SEE HOW THINGS FIT NOW WITH A BIG BELLY AND BIGGER BOOBS!

IT WON'T HAPPEN EVERY DAY, BUT WHEN YOU FEEL LIKE IT, FLAUNT IT! PREGNANT BODIES ARE ICONIC!

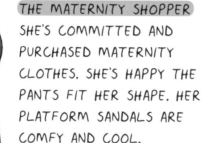

WHY ARE SO MANY MATERNITY CLOTHES STRIPED?

Maternity

THE MATERNITY SHOPPER

SHE'S COMMITTED AND PURCHASED MATERNITY CLOTHES. SHE'S HAPPY THE PANTS FIT HER SHAPE. HER PLATFORM SANDALS ARE COMFY AND COOL.

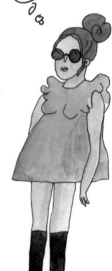

I DO NOT WANT TO IDENTIFY AS PREGNANT TODAY.

THE MYSTERY DRESSER

SHE'S FEELING NAUSEOUS AND BLOATED ON THE INSIDE, BUT ON THE OUTSIDE SHE LOOKS FABULOUS. THE DARK SUNGLASSES SAY "DON'T TALK TO ME."

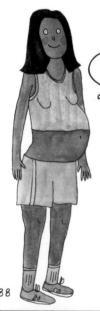

MAYBE I'LL STRETCH LATER...

ATHLEISURE ALL THE WAY

SHE'S REALLY COMFY IN HER SHORTS AND TANK WITH THE BELLY HANGING OUT. MATCHING CUSHY GYM SHOES COMPLETE THE OUTFIT.

Styles

I THINK MY NEWBORN WILL FIT IN HERE WITH ME.

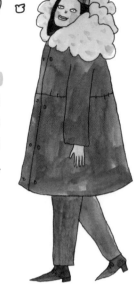

BIG COAT

SHE DOESN'T CARE IF HER BELLY IS VISIBLE OR NOT, SHE'S JUST HAPPY TO BE COZY AND WARM WITH HER ONE-SIZE-LARGER COAT.

NOW WHERE DID I LEAVE MY SNACK?

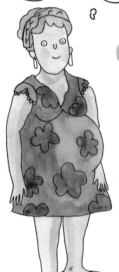

THE SAME

SHE'S LITERALLY WEARING THE SAME DRESS AND SANDALS SHE WOULD BE WEARING ANYWAYS. THIS TIME THE BELLY IS JUST STRETCHING A BIT MORE THAN NORMAL.

MUHAHAHAHAHA!

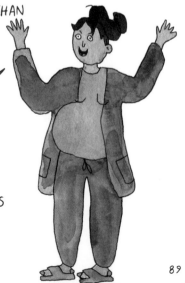

SWEATS QUEEN

LITERALLY AS COMFORTABLE AS HUMANLY POSSIBLE.

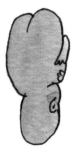

BABY POSITIONS

THE BABY HAS FEW WAYS OF EXPRESSING HERSELF AT THIS POINT. ONE OF THOSE WAYS IS HOW SHE CHOOSES TO POSITION HERSELF. THE MOST OPPORTUNE WAY FOR BABY TO BE POSITIONED FOR BIRTH IS FACING YOUR BACK AND FACE DOWN (OCCIPUT ANTERIOR). SHE COULD ALSO BE SIDEWAYS (TRANSVERSE), FACING YOUR FRONT (POSTERIOR), AND OF COURSE UPRIGHT (BREECH).

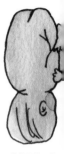

ANTERIOR

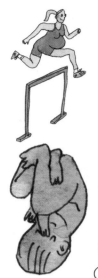

POSTERIOR

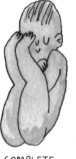

COMPLETE BREECH

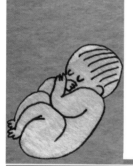

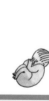

25% OF BABIES ARE BREECH AT 28 WEEKS.

7% AT 32 WEEKS

3–4% AT FULL TERM

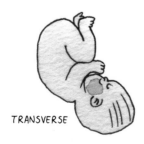

INCOMPLETE BREECH

ANTERIOR

TRANSVERSE

FRANK BREECH

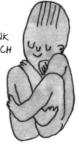

TRANSVERSE

THE PLACENTA

THE BABY ISN'T THE ONLY ORGANISM INSIDE YOU THAT CAN BE IN
DIFFERENT POSITIONS, AND I'M NOT TALKING ABOUT DAD. THE
PLACENTA IS A LITERAL ORGAN THAT YOU CREATE ALONG WITH
BABY. IT MAKES SURE THAT BABY IS GETTING OXYGEN AND
NUTRIENTS, AND IT REMOVES WASTE.

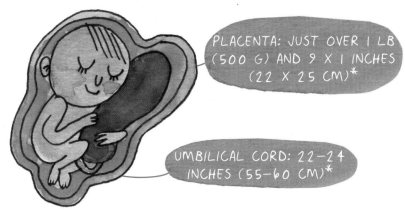

PLACENTA: JUST OVER 1 LB
(500 G) AND 9 X 1 INCHES
(22 X 25 CM)*

UMBILICAL CORD: 22-24
INCHES (55-60 CM)*

THE PLACENTA CAN BE ANYWHERE AROUND THE BABY, NORMALLY
ON THE TOP OR SIDE OF YOUR UTERUS. SOMETIMES IT'S IN FRONT
OF YOUR BABY (ANTERIOR PLACENTA) SO IT CAN MAKE KICKS A
BIT HARDER TO FEEL. IF THE PLACENTA IS TOO LOW (PLACENTA
PREVIA) YOUR DOCTOR WILL LET YOU KNOW. THIS HAPPENS IN
ABOUT 0.5% OF PREGNANCIES.

*SIZE AND WEIGHT ARE AVERAGES AT BIRTH.

YOU PROBABLY LOOK PREGNANT BY NOW

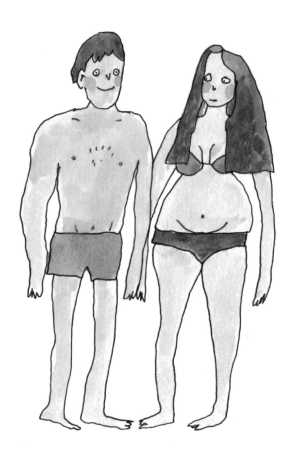

AS YOUR BODY CHANGES (GETS BIGGER), YOU HAVE NOTICED YOUR PARTNER'S DAD BOD CHANGING TOO. HE'S ACTUALLY GOTTEN FITTER AS TIME GOES ON! FEELS LIKE THE 21 POUNDS YOU'VE GAINED HAVE COME DIRECTLY FROM HIM!

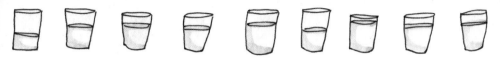

DRINK WATER

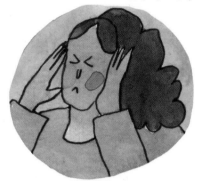

HEADACHE? WATER

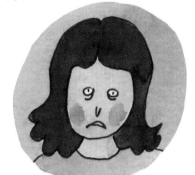

NAUSEOUS? WATER

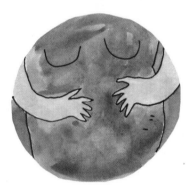

SORTA HUNGRY BUT
FEEL TOO FULL? WATER

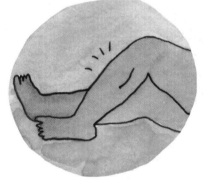

LEG CRAMPS? WATER

WATER IS CRUCIAL RIGHT NOW. YOUR BLOOD VOLUME IS DOUBLING, YOU
ARE GROWING A BABY AND A PLACENTA AS WELL AS ALL THE FLUID
SURROUNDING THEM—PLUS ALL THE WATER YOU NORMALLY NEED.
WATER CAN ALSO BE A QUICK AND EASY FIX.

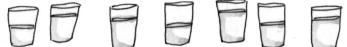

DISCLAIMER: WATER IS NOT GUARANTEED TO FIX ANY OR ALL OF YOUR
PROBLEMS, BUT IT DOESN'T HURT TO TRY IT!

The Birthing

BIRTHING PHILOSOPHIES ARE ON A SPECTRUM, AND CHANCES ARE YOU PROBABLY SEE YOURSELF IN THE MIDDLE OF THE TWO POLARITIES. BUT SOMEHOW IT FEELS LIKE YOU SHOULD CONFORM TO ONE OR THE OTHER. THIS IS BECAUSE MANY OF THE LOUDEST VOICES IN BIRTHING ARE THE ONES THAT HAVE THE STRONGEST VIEWS.

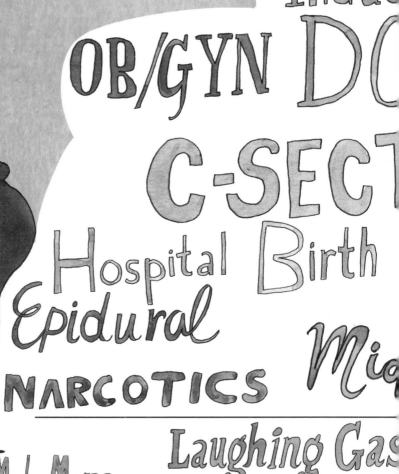

Induc

OB/GYN DC

C-SECT

Hospital Birth

Epidural

NARCOTICS Mi

Laughing Gas

Modern Meds Mama

HOWEVER, IF YOU HAVE NEVER DONE THIS, IT'S OK IF YOU DON'T HAVE STRONG FEELINGS OR YOU WANT A MIX OF TREATMENTS OR YOU DON'T KNOW EXACTLY WHAT YOU WANT. JUST TAKE TIME TO LEARN ABOUT YOUR OPTIONS AND GO WITH YOUR GUT AND THE MEDICAL ADVICE YOU RECEIVE FROM PROFESSIONALS. AND IF YOU KNOW WHAT YOU WANT, THEN GO FOR IT!

on

JLA

ON

"Natural" Birth

HOME BIRTH

ORGASMIC BIRTH

rife

Hypnobirthing

Hippie Mommie

Relaxing
while pregnant

IT'S OBVIOUS THAT YOUR BODY IS DOING
A LOT OF WORK, AND YOUR APPETITE
SUPPORTS THIS, BUT ALSO SO ARE YOU!
YOU ARE REALLY BUSY RIGHT NOW
CREATING LIFE 24 HOURS A DAY, SEVEN
DAYS A WEEK.

SO, PART OF YOUR JOB IS TO MAKE
SURE YOU GET THAT NICE CHILL TIME.
THE FOLLOWING SECTION GIVES IDEAS
AND RECOMMENDATIONS (AND MAKES
SPACE) FOR THIS MUCH-NEEDED
RELAXATION.

WALKING IS A GREAT WAY TO RELAX, AND THERE ARE STUDIES THAT SAY
THAT WOMEN WHO WERE ACTIVE DURING PREGNANCY HAVE SHORTER
LABORS. IF YOU'RE ABLE, A DAILY WALK IS AN EASY WAY TO GET THE
BLOOD MOVING AND IS FABULOUS FOR MENTAL HEALTH AS WELL.

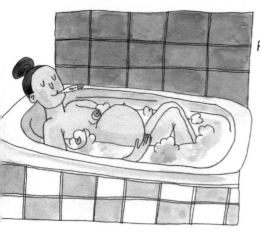

BATHS CAN FEEL AMAZING WHILE PREGNANT. EXPERTS WARN TO KEEP YOUR TEMPERATURE UNDER 102 DEGREES FAHRENHEIT (39 C). IF YOU'RE WORRIED YOU'RE GETTING TOO HOT YOU CAN BRING A THERMOMETER TO TAKE YOUR TEMPERATURE IN THE TUB.

THE BODY PILLOW LOOKS RIDICULOUS. BUT IT'S ALL OVER THE INTERNET FOR A REASON.

YOGA STRETCHES CAN ALLEVIATE MANY ACHES AND PAINS THAT ARE COMMON IN PREGNANCY.

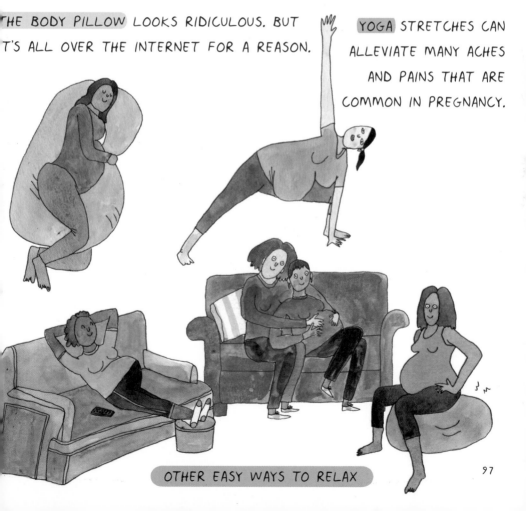

OTHER EASY WAYS TO RELAX

"EASY" PREGNANCIES ARE STILL PREGNANCIES

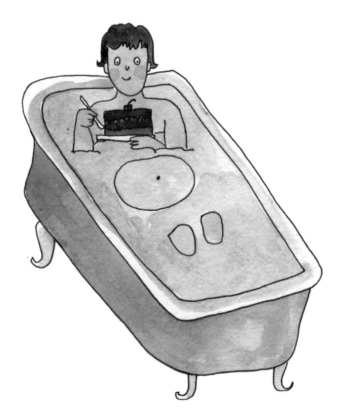

THE SIXTH MONTH SEEMED TO GO THE FASTEST SO FAR. YOU ATE
LOTS OF DESSERTS AND YOU'RE FEELING MOSTLY GOOD. SOME DAYS
ARE TOUGH AND IT HELPS TO TAKE IT EASY AND TAKE BATHS.
ALTHOUGH YOU FEEL AS THOUGH YOU HAD AN "EASIER" PREGNANCY,
AS IN NO COMPLICATIONS AND DECENT ENERGY AS WELL AS GOOD
SUPPORT SYSTEM AND WORK SCHEDULE, IT'S STILL HARD.

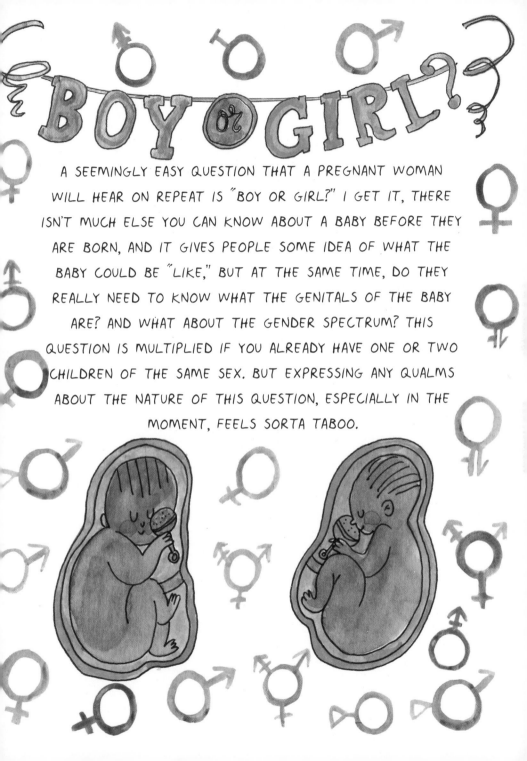

BOY or GIRL?

A SEEMINGLY EASY QUESTION THAT A PREGNANT WOMAN WILL HEAR ON REPEAT IS "BOY OR GIRL?" I GET IT, THERE ISN'T MUCH ELSE YOU CAN KNOW ABOUT A BABY BEFORE THEY ARE BORN, AND IT GIVES PEOPLE SOME IDEA OF WHAT THE BABY COULD BE "LIKE," BUT AT THE SAME TIME, DO THEY REALLY NEED TO KNOW WHAT THE GENITALS OF THE BABY ARE? AND WHAT ABOUT THE GENDER SPECTRUM? THIS QUESTION IS MULTIPLIED IF YOU ALREADY HAVE ONE OR TWO CHILDREN OF THE SAME SEX. BUT EXPRESSING ANY QUALMS ABOUT THE NATURE OF THIS QUESTION, ESPECIALLY IN THE MOMENT, FEELS SORTA TABOO.

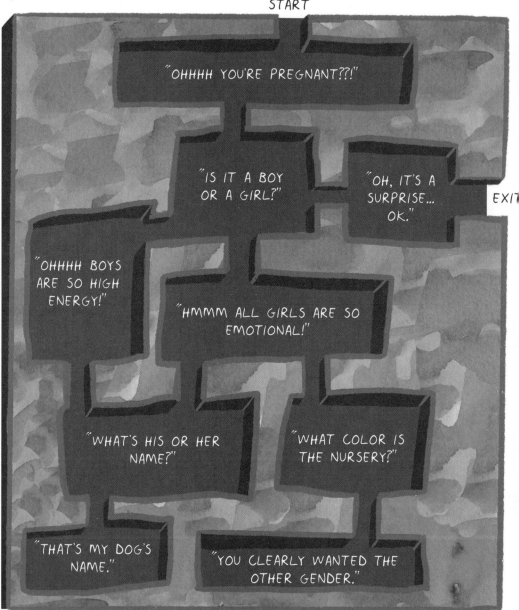

"Gender" Questions Maze

START

"OHHHH YOU'RE PREGNANT???!"

"IS IT A BOY OR A GIRL?"

"OH, IT'S A SURPRISE... OK."

EXIT

"OHHHH BOYS ARE SO HIGH ENERGY!"

"HMMM ALL GIRLS ARE SO EMOTIONAL!"

"WHAT'S HIS OR HER NAME?"

"WHAT COLOR IS THE NURSERY?"

"THAT'S MY DOG'S NAME."

"YOU CLEARLY WANTED THE OTHER GENDER."

(EXAMPLES ABOVE ARE TRUE TO LIFE AND IN NO WAY REFLECT THE VIEWPOINTS OF THE AUTHOR.)

THE GENDER REVEAL

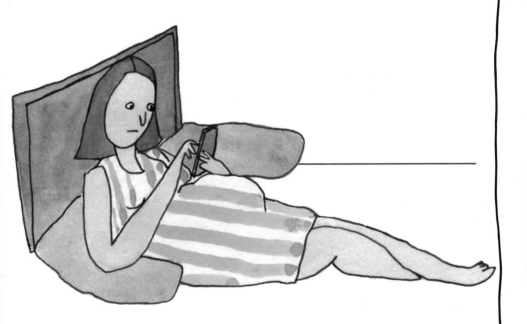

YOUR BABY SHOWER IS COMING UP AND YOU HAVE KEPT THE SEX OF THE BABY A SURPRISE TO YOUR FRIENDS AND FAMILY UNTIL NOW, BUT WANT TO REVEAL IT AT THE PARTY. HOWEVER, ALL YOUR GOOGLING TURNS UP VERY TRADITIONAL GENDER REVEALS (AND FIRES!), AND YOU'RE NOT REALLY A TRADITIONAL GAL (AND DON'T WANT TO START A FOREST FIRE).

YOU THINK OF AN ORIGINAL IDEA, BUT PRETEND LIKE YOU'RE GOING TO DO THE REVEAL THROUGH A PINK OR BLUE CAKE CUT, WHICH IS A FINE WAY TO DO IT. ANY WAY THAT DOESN'T START A FIRE IS A GOOD WAY, IT'S JUST NOT REALLY "YOU."

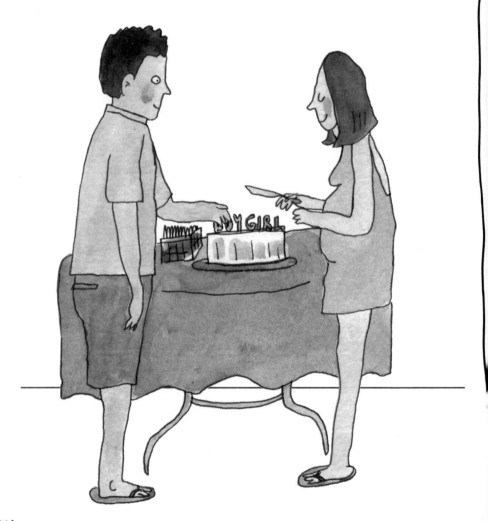

JUST WHEN YOU'RE ABOUT TO CUT THE CAKE, YOU AND YOUR HUSBAND MOON THE PARTY WITH BLUE MARKS ON YOUR BUTTS! GASPS, LAUGHS, AND CHEERS ENSUE. A VERY ORIGINAL GENDER REVEAL, INDEED. EVERYONE IS SO SHOCKED THAT THEY FORGET TO TELL YOU WHAT "THE DIFFERENCES ARE" BETWEEN BOYS AND GIRLS.

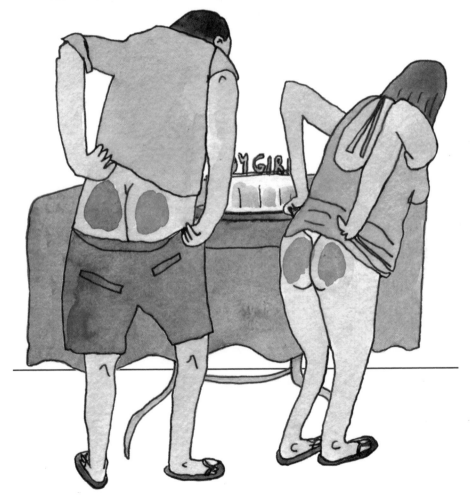

WHAT WILL BABY LOOK LIKE?
FANTASIZING ABOUT THE FUTURE

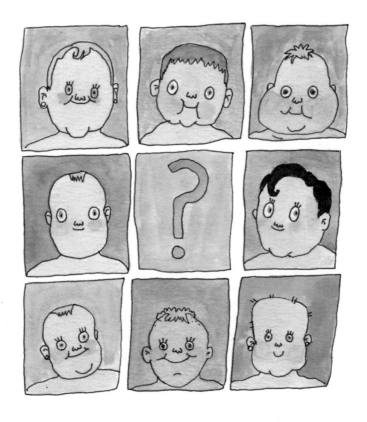

NO MATTER WHAT THE BABY'S SEX IS, THE MOST IMPORTANT THING IS
THAT THE BABY IS HEALTHY—BUT IT'S FUN TO THINK ABOUT WHAT THE
BABY WILL LOOK LIKE WHEN HE IS BORN. WILL HE HAVE MOMMY'S EYES?
WILL HE HAVE DADDY'S HAIR? WILL HE EVEN HAVE HAIR? BIG CHIN? WILL
HE LOOK LIKE THE BABY IN YOUR DREAM? ONLY TIME WILL TELL. ALL
WE KNOW FOR CERTAIN IS THAT HE WILL BE ADORABLE.

Sex
WHILE PREGNANT

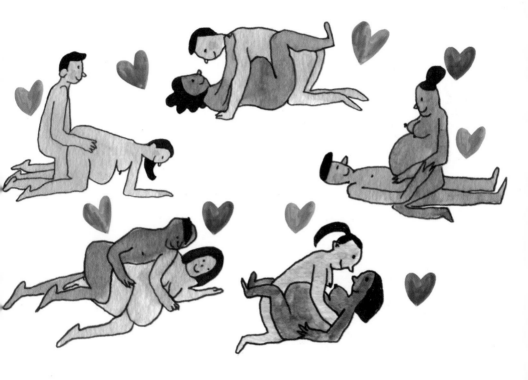

SPEAKING ABOUT SEX, UNLESS YOUR DOCTOR HAS TOLD YOU OTHERWISE, SEX HAS BEEN SHOWN TO BE GREAT FOR A PREGNANT WOMAN. SOME SAY IT HELPS SHORTEN LABOR AND HELPS LABOR START CLOSER TO FORTY WEEKS, WHILE OTHERS SAY IF IT FEELS GOOD, DO IT. ONE STRANGE THING ABOUT SEX AT THIS STAGE IS THE DIFFERENT ANGLES YOU HAVE TO GET IN TO GET IT IN. I GUESS IT'S AN EXCUSE TO GET CREATIVE?

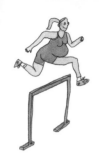

THE GLUCOSE TEST

HAPPENS BETWEEN 24–28 WEEKS

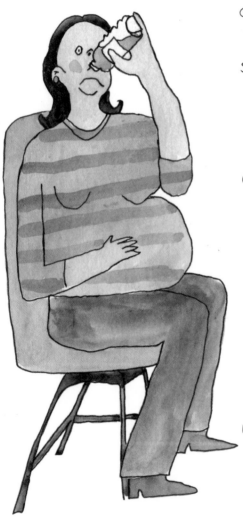

THE GLUCOSE TEST SCREENS FOR GESTATIONAL DIABETES. IT SEEMS LIKE THE EASIEST TEST. JUST DRINK A SUGARY DRINK, THEN GET YOUR BLOOD DRAWN. HOWEVER, SINCE IT'S LIKE PURPOSEFULLY GIVING YOURSELF A SUGAR RUSH, THE TEST IS ACTUALLY QUITE EXHAUSTING. BECAUSE MANY OF THE SYMPTOMS FOR GESTATIONAL DIABETES (THIRST, HUNGER, FATIGUE) ARE NORMAL PREGNANCY SYMPTOMS, THERE IS NO WAY TO KNOW IF YOU HAVE IT BEFORE THE TEST. THE IMPORTANT THING IS YOU'LL SOON BE FINDING OUT. IF YOU TEST POSITIVE, YOUR DOCTOR WILL HELP MAKE SURE THAT YOU AND YOUR BABY STAY AS HEALTHY AS POSSIBLE.

PREGNANCY IN
The Movies vs. in Reality

PREGNANCY IN THE MOVIES: A WOMAN THROWS UP ONCE IN THE MORNING, TAKES A PREGNANCY TEST IMMEDIATELY AFTER, AND SPENDS THE REST OF THE PREGNANCY WALKING AROUND CAREFREE AND GLOWING.

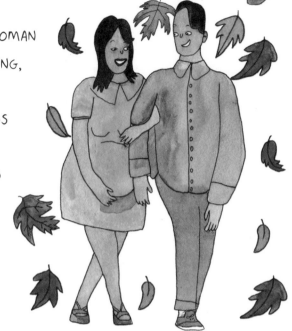

IN REAL LIFE: A PREGNANT WOMAN SITS AND KEEPS GOOGLING STRANGE SYMPTOMS THAT SHE NEVER ASSOCIATED WITH PREGNANCY AND KEEPS FINDING OUT THAT YES, THEY ARE TOTALLY NORMAL.

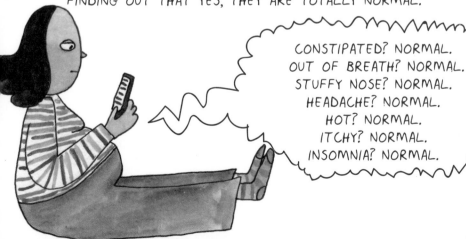

CONSTIPATED? NORMAL.
OUT OF BREATH? NORMAL.
STUFFY NOSE? NORMAL.
HEADACHE? NORMAL.
HOT? NORMAL.
ITCHY? NORMAL.
INSOMNIA? NORMAL.

Second Trimester

BY THE END OF THE SECOND TRIMESTER YOU WILL LIKELY HAVE
ACCOMPLISHED THE FOLLOWING:

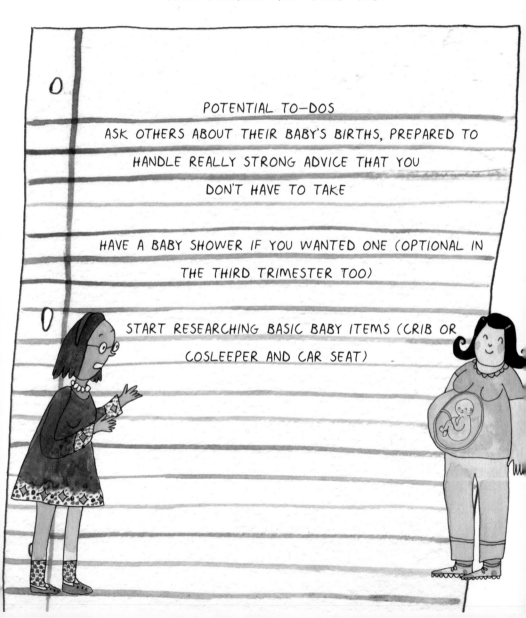

POTENTIAL TO-DOS

ASK OTHERS ABOUT THEIR BABY'S BIRTHS, PREPARED TO
HANDLE REALLY STRONG ADVICE THAT YOU
DON'T HAVE TO TAKE

HAVE A BABY SHOWER IF YOU WANTED ONE (OPTIONAL IN
THE THIRD TRIMESTER TOO)

START RESEARCHING BASIC BABY ITEMS (CRIB OR
COSLEEPER AND CAR SEAT)

Third Trimester

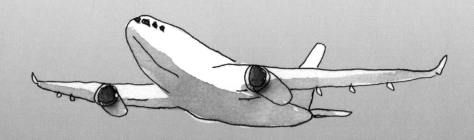

GETTING READY
FOR LIFTOFF

Prepping for Birth

PREPARING FOR LABOR AND THE BIRTH OF YOUR BABY CAN FEEL LIKE BEING THE PILOT OF A FLIGHT.

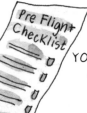

YOU CREATE A CHECKLIST (BIRTH PLAN AND/OR ITEMS TO BRING).

YOU PACK A BAG.

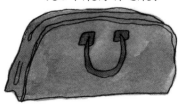

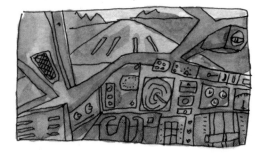

YOU IMAGINE AND LIKELY PRACTICE THE "SCENARIO."

ONLY YOU ARE CAPABLE OF FLYING (BIRTHING) THE METAPHORICAL PLANE (BABY).

A COPILOT (DOCTOR) IS THERE SHOULD YOU NEED ASSISTANCE.

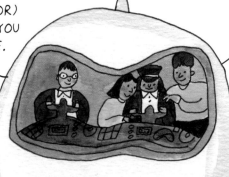

PREPPING CAN BE ANYTHING YOU WANT

YOU DO SOME RESEARCH ON WHAT YOU MIGHT NEED FOR BIRTH AND POSTPARTUM AND YOU DECIDE TO TREAT YOURSELF WITH A TRIP TO THE FANCY HEALTH FOOD STORE.

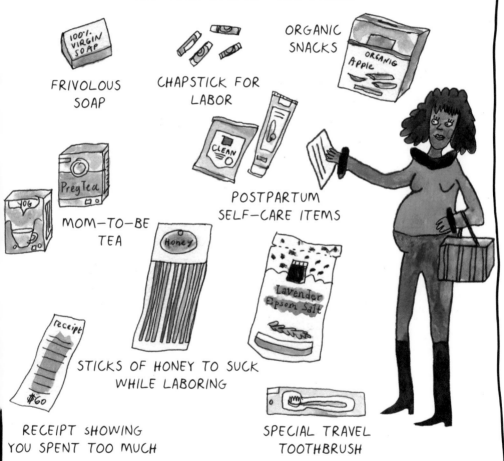

FRIVOLOUS SOAP

CHAPSTICK FOR LABOR

ORGANIC SNACKS

MOM-TO-BE TEA

POSTPARTUM SELF-CARE ITEMS

STICKS OF HONEY TO SUCK WHILE LABORING

RECEIPT SHOWING YOU SPENT TOO MUCH

SPECIAL TRAVEL TOOTHBRUSH

IT'S A FUN, RELAXING, AND LOW-STAKES ACTIVITY WHEN THINGS ARE FEELING LIKE THEY ARE GETTING SERIOUS—PLUS, CAPITALISM!

The 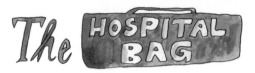 HOSPITAL BAG

JUST LIKE FRIVOLOUS SPENDING CAN BRING COMFORT TO SOME, SO TOO CAN PACKING A HOSPITAL BAG. FOR THOSE WHO FIND THIS ACTIVITY STRESSFUL, THE GOOD NEWS IS, YOU'RE BUILT WITH EVERYTHING YOU NEED TO DELIVER YOUR BABY, SO THE PRESSURE SHOULD BE AS LOW AS PACKING A WEEKEND BAG.

THE BASICS

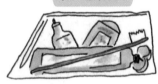

A TOOTHBRUSH, SHAMPOO/ CONDITIONER, SOAP, BRUSH, PHONE CHARGERS, HAIR TIES, ETC.

SNACKS

FOR YOU AND YOUR PARTNER, FOR LABOR (IF ALLOWED) AND AFTERWARDS.

COMFY CLOTHES

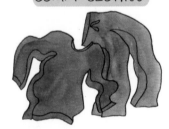

YOUR BUMP IS STILL AROUND AFTER BABY IS BORN, SO COMFY CLOTHES ARE A MUST. ALSO, YOUR HORMONES WILL LIKELY MESS WITH YOUR INTERNAL TEMP, SO BRING LAYERS.

COMFORT ACTIVITIES

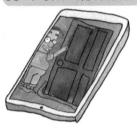

THIS COULD BE A BOOK, YOUR IPAD WITH A SPECIAL MOVIE/TV SHOW, KNITTING, OR ANYTHING ELSE YOU FIND COMFORTING TO DO WHILE YOU WAIT OR HANG AT THE HOSPITAL.

FOR BABY: YOU WON'T NEED MUCH FOR BABY EXCEPT FOR A CAR SEAT IF YOU'RE DRIVING HOME AND A "GOING HOME" OUTFIT FOR WHEN THE BABY LEAVES THE HOSPITAL.

The Body

WHILE YOU ARE GETTING READY TO BIRTH YOUR BABY, SO IS YOUR BODY. DEPENDING ON YOUR PREPREGNANCY WEIGHT, YOU'LL BE ADVISED TO GAIN BETWEEN 11 AND 40 POUNDS.

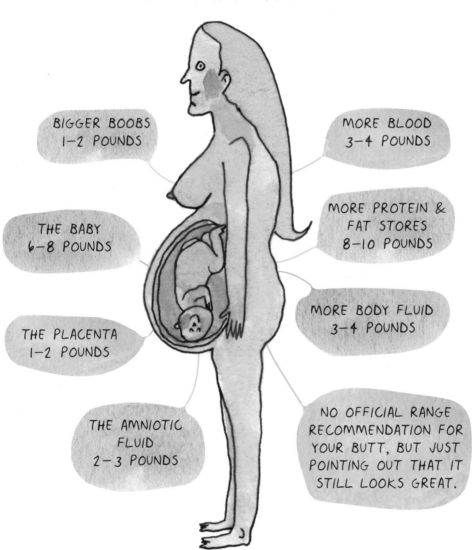

BIGGER BOOBS
1-2 POUNDS

MORE BLOOD
3-4 POUNDS

THE BABY
6-8 POUNDS

MORE PROTEIN &
FAT STORES
8-10 POUNDS

THE PLACENTA
1-2 POUNDS

MORE BODY FLUID
3-4 POUNDS

THE AMNIOTIC
FLUID
2-3 POUNDS

NO OFFICIAL RANGE
RECOMMENDATION FOR
YOUR BUTT, BUT JUST
POINTING OUT THAT IT
STILL LOOKS GREAT.

At Seven Months

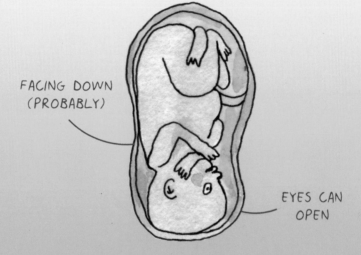

FACING DOWN
(PROBABLY)

EYES CAN
OPEN

WEEKS
28–31

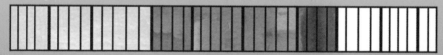

EVERY DAY IS A WORKOUT WHEN YOU'RE SEVEN
MONTHS PREGNANT. ON YOUR DAYS OFF YOU
MIGHT SLEEP IN AND THEN TAKE A MORNING
NAP AND, LATER, AN AFTERNOON NAP.

AVERAGE END-OF-MONTH SIZE: 16.18 IN (41.1 CM)

Third-Trimester Feelings

THE DUE DATE: NOW THAT YOU'RE IN THE FINAL STRETCH, YOU MAY START TO NOTICE FUTURE DATES AND COMPARE THEM TO YOUR ESTIMATED DUE DATE.

THE BELLY: EVEN THOUGH IT HAS BEEN A GRADUAL CHANGE, AND THERE'S A BEAUTIFUL BABY INSIDE IT, THE BELLY MAY STILL TAKE SOME GETTING USED TO. ONE WAY TO OWN THIS CHANGE IS TO GIVE IT A NICKNAME. IT GIVES YOU MORE CONTROL OVER IT.

CONFLICTING EMOTIONS: AT THIS POINT YOU MAY BE FEELING RELIEVED THAT YOU HAVE MADE IT THIS FAR! YOU MAY ALSO BE FEELING ANTICIPATION FOR THE BIG DAY.

ESTIMATED DUE DATE

SPEAKING OF DUE DATES, ESTIMATED DUE DATES ARE JUST THAT, AN ESTIMATION. IT'S JUST SUCH A WIDE NET REALLY, LIKE AN ENTIRE MONTH WHERE IT'S NORMAL TO HAVE YOUR BABY. TWO PEOPLE MIGHT HAVE THE EXACT SAME DUE DATE, BUT HAVE THEIR BABIES THREE WEEKS APART, AND IT WOULD STILL BE A NORMAL RANGE.

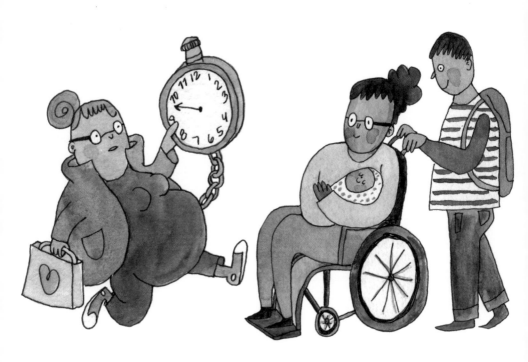

ONLY TIME WILL TELL

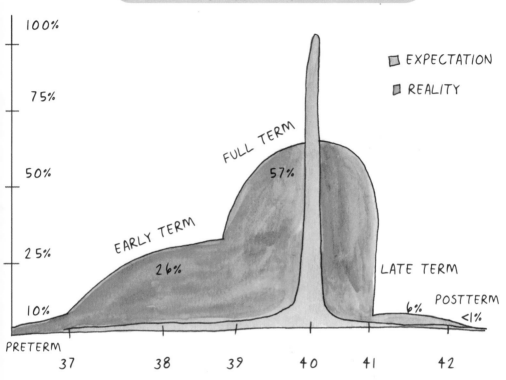

A DUE DATE IS CALCULATED BY YOUR LAST PERIOD PLUS 280 DAYS. IT ASSUMES ALL PERIOD CYCLES ARE 28 DAYS AND THAT WE ALL OVULATE ON THE 14TH DAY. BOTH OF THESE ARE JUST ESTIMATIONS AND THERE-FORE, LOGICALLY, ONLY ABOUT 3% OF WOMEN ACTUALLY GIVE BIRTH ON THEIR DUE DATE.

ABOUT THE GRAPH: EACH NUMBER IS THE NUMBER OF WEEKS AND ZERO DAYS. THE DATA INCLUDE C-SECTIONS AND INDUCTIONS.

Sleeping

THE NIGHTTIME PUZZLE

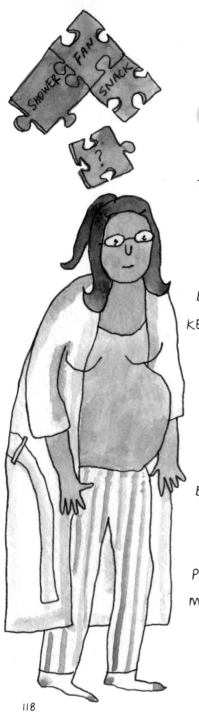

SNOOZING CAN BE TOUGH IN THE THIRD TRIMESTER (ALL TRIMESTERS?), AND GETTING COMFORTABLE ENOUGH TO SLEEP MAY FEEL LIKE A NIGHTLY PUZZLE. DON'T LET PEOPLE BULLY YOU ABOUT GETTING NO SLEEP WHEN BABY COMES. YES, IT'S TRUE A NEWBORN WILL KEEP NEW PARENTS UP, BUT YOU'LL HAVE A CUTE LITTLE NEWBORN TO GET UP FOR!

THE THIRD TRIMESTER CAN BE PARTICULARLY DIFFICULT BECAUSE BABY'S BIGGER, SO YOUR BLADDER (AND EVERYTHING ELSE) IS SQUISHED.

ALSO, THERE'S SOME SORT OF PREGNANCY-RELATED INSOMNIA (I DON'T KNOW, MAYBE YOU'RE ANXIOUS BECAUSE SOON YOU'LL BE BIRTHING A HUMAN???).

PILLOWS ARE PART OF THE SOLUTION

THERE'S A STRONG CHANCE YOU MIGHT START TO RELATE MORE TO YOUR OLDER COWORKERS OR FRIENDS WHO HAVE BACK AND HIP ISSUES AND HAVE TROUBLE SLEEPING. AT LEAST YOU KNOW YOUR TROUBLES WILL PROBABLY GO AWAY ONCE YOU HAVE THAT BABY! PILLOWS ARE GREAT FOR GETTING COMFY IN THE LAST TRIMESTER. SOME WOMEN EVEN SLEEP IN A SEPARATE BED FROM THEIR PARTNER FOR A WHILE TO HAVE MORE SPACE. NO SHAME IN THAT.

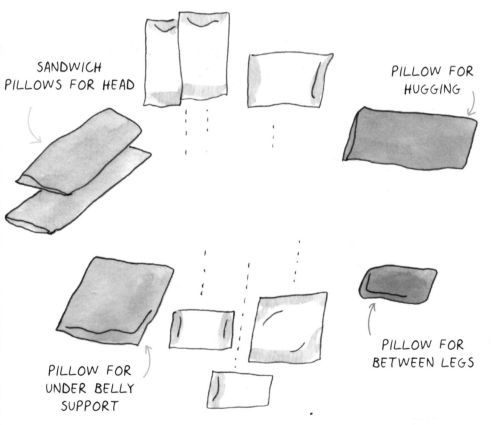

SANDWICH PILLOWS FOR HEAD

PILLOW FOR HUGGING

PILLOW FOR UNDER BELLY SUPPORT

PILLOW FOR BETWEEN LEGS

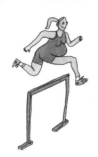

THE MOVEMENT!!!

LIKELY BY 30TH WEEK

ENOUGH ABOUT SLEEP, LET'S TALK ABOUT THAT BELLY! AT SOME POINT IN THE LATER WEEKS OF PREGNANCY, MANY WOMEN WILL SEE THEIR BABY FROM THE OUTSIDE! IT'S AN EXTRAORDINARY AND TRULY AMAZING SIGHT TO SEE! NOW YOUR LOVED ONES GET A VISUAL TASTE OF THEIR NEW FAMILY MEMBER WITH THEIR OWN "HUNGRY-FOR-BABY" EYES.

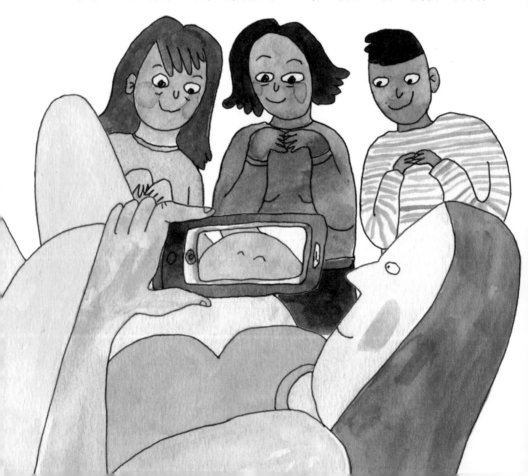

The Comments

BY THE THIRD TRIMESTER YOU WILL LIKELY LOOK UNQUESTIONABLY PREGNANT. READ: BELLY IS OUT THERE. THIS TENDS TO GET PEOPLE EXCITED. EVEN THOUGH THEY HAVE NO BUSINESS COMMENTING, COMMENTS ARE UNAVOIDABLE AND OFTEN CONFLICTING.

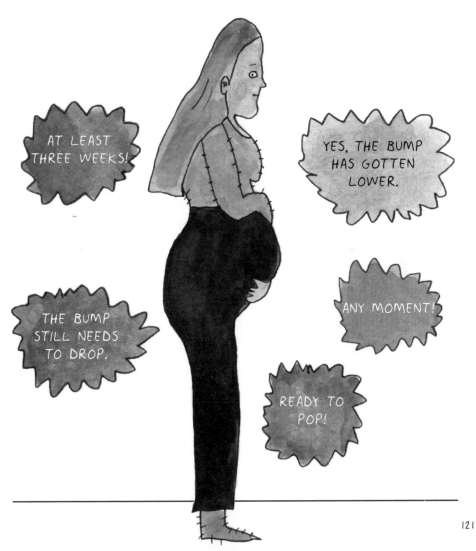

Canned Responses

IN FACT, YOU'LL LIKELY HEAR SOME OF THE FOLLOWING. I'VE PREPPED SOME CANNED RESPONSES FOR YOU SO YOU DON'T HAVE TO SMILE AND NOD IF YOU DON'T WANT TO. ADDED VALUE: A HELPFUL CHART FOR ANYONE WHO PLANS TO MAKE ANY OF THESE COMMENTS...

COMMENT	WHY IT'S FRUSTRATING	CANNED RESPONSE
"SLEEP NOW WHILE YOU CAN!"	TELLING SOMEONE TO SLEEP WHEN THEY CAN'T AND WISH THEY COULD IS VEXING AT MILDEST. ADD A BIG BELLY AND THE MIDNIGHT PEE BREAKS AND REALIZE THE COMMENT IS ACTUALLY PRETTY CRUEL.	"WOW, YOU JUST SAID THE MOST TYPICAL COMMENT AIMED AT PREGNANT LADIES! COOL."
"YOUR BELLY LOOKS LIKE [INSERT ANY OBJECT HERE]."	UNLESS YOU NAILED EXACTLY WHAT THE PREGNANT LADY FEELS LIKE HER BELLY LOOKS LIKE AT THE MOMENT, YOU ARE WRONG. AND REALLY, THERE IS NO BENEFIT IN YOU TELLING HER WHAT HER BODY LOOKS LIKE TO YOU—JUST LIKE ANY PERSON'S BODY, SURPRISE!	"HA HA HA HA HA..."
"YOU'LL BE ALL STRETCHED OUT FOR THE SECOND ONE!"	ARE YOU REALLY COMMENTING ON SOMEONE'S VAGINA AND/OR OTHER BODY PARTS AND HOW THEY ARE GOING TO BE STRETCHED OUT? ALSO, LET'S FOCUS ON THE BABY AT HAND AND NOT A HYPOTHETICAL ONE.	A SILENT GLARE IS A GOOD RESPONSE HERE. (MAYBE THEY'LL USE THAT TIME TO THINK ABOUT WHAT THEY SAID.)

COMMENT	WHY IT'S FRUSTRATING	CANNED RESPONSE
"WOW! YOUR BELLY IS ENORMOUS! IT'S GETTING SO BIG, ETC, ETC."	SAY IT WITH ME—DO NOT COMMENT ON ANY WOMAN'S BODY—PERIOD!	"YES, THAT'S WHAT IT'S SUPPOSED TO DO IN THERE. IT WOULD BE WEIRD IF IT STOPPED GROWING..."
"YOU'LL PROBABLY GO INTO LABOR LATE/EARLY."	THAT'S ACTUALLY NOT TRUE. SERIOUSLY KEEP YOUR (INVALID) PREDICTIONS TO YOURSELF, THEY AREN'T DOING ANYONE ANY FAVORS. ONLY TIME WILL TELL, NOT YOU.	"YUP, IT'S REALLY GONNA BE CHANCE."
"YOU CAN'T HAVE JUST ONE!"	HAVING A BABY IS A BIG DEAL. THAT IS POTENTIALLY HAPPENING FOR THE FIRST TIME. MAYBE I ONLY WANT ONE, OR MAYBE I'LL ONLY HAVE ONE. IN ANY CASE, THIS IS REALLY AN INSIDE THOUGHT.	"ACTUALLY, I CAN JUST HAVE ONE."

TO SUMMARIZE, A LOT OF THE TIME, PEOPLE DON'T THINK BEFORE THEY SPEAK AND JUST SAY THE FIRST THING THAT COMES INTO THEIR HEAD. YOU DON'T HAVE TO ACCEPT WHAT THEY SAY OR RESPOND AT ALL. SOMETIMES JUST NODDING AND SAYING "WE'LL SEE" DOES THE TRICK. IN THE END, IT'S REALLY JUST EMBARRASSING FOR THEM THAT THEY CAN'T COME UP WITH SOMETHING BETTER TO SAY TO YOU.

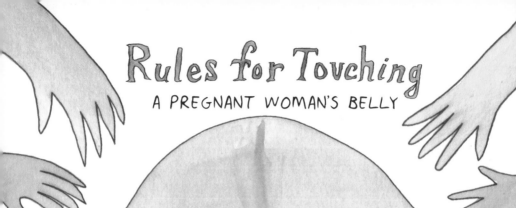

Rules for Touching
A PREGNANT WOMAN'S BELLY

1) ONLY TOUCH IF SHE OFFERS. IF YOU'RE DYING TO TOUCH HER, PLEASE ASK, AND BE PREPARED TO BE TOLD NO.

2) DON'T ASK TO TOUCH WHILE YOU'RE ALREADY REACHING OVER TO TOUCH OR ALREADY TOUCHING HER. THAT'S RUDE.

3) DON'T TRY TO TOUCH IT WHEN IT'S REALLY NOT EVEN A BELLY YET.

4) TOUCH GENTLY, RESPECTFULLY, AND WITH ONE HAND.

5) DON'T PAT IT.

6) AND DON'T SAY "MY BABY" WHILE PATTING IT.

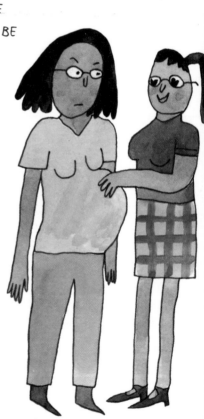

STRANGER SURPRISE

YOU HAD HEARD HORROR STORIES OF STRANGERS TOUCHING BELLIES AND GIVING UNSOLICITED ADVICE. AND FINALLY, WELL INTO YOUR THIRD TRIMESTER, A STRANGER ASKS IF YOU ARE PREGNANT (LOL).

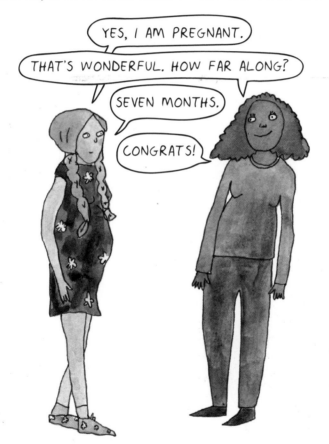

YES, I AM PREGNANT.

THAT'S WONDERFUL. HOW FAR ALONG?

SEVEN MONTHS.

CONGRATS!

IT IS ACTUALLY A TOTALLY NORMAL INTERACTION. SHE DIDN'T COMMENT ON YOUR BODY OR ASK INTRUSIVE QUESTIONS. SHE WAS GENUINELY HAPPY FOR YOU. YOU FEEL THANKFUL.

THE SPOTLIGHT IS ON THEM

YOU ARE AT THE GYM. AFTER YOU ARE DONE WORKING OUT, A NICE OLDER LADY YOU'VE SEEN AROUND MANY TIMES TALKS TO YOU FOR THE FIRST TIME.

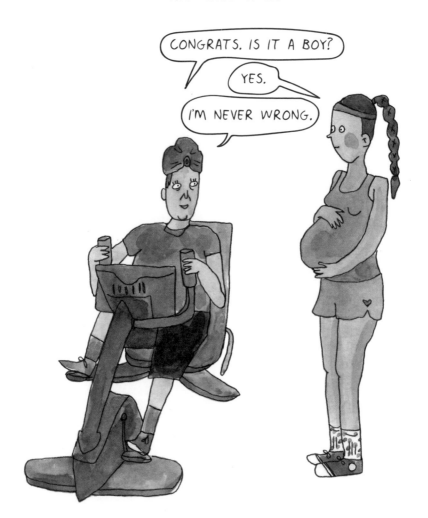

YOU DON'T RESPOND

YOU ARE ON A WALK WITH YOUR PARTNER. AN OLDER WOMAN YELLS FROM A BENCH.

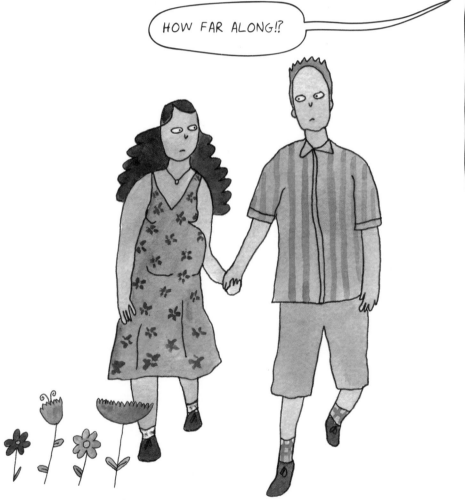

HOW FAR ALONG!?

YOU IGNORE HER AND KEEP WALKING.

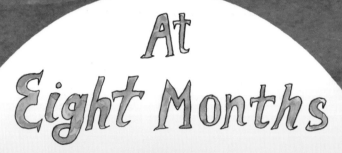

At Eight Months

MOVING OFTEN

BRAIN CONTINUING TO DEVELOP

GETTING EVEN MORE FAT—I MEAN CUTE!

WEEKS
32 – 36

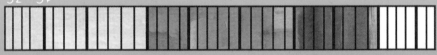

PHYSICALLY, THE EIGHTH MONTH CAN BE TOUGH. THE BABY IS CRUSHING YOUR INNARDS AND YOU GOTTA PEE ALL THE TIME. EMOTIONALLY, IT'S DEFINITELY A MIXED BAG—YOU ARE SO CLOSE!

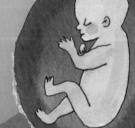

AVERAGE END-OF-MONTH SIZE: 18.66 IN (47.4 CM)

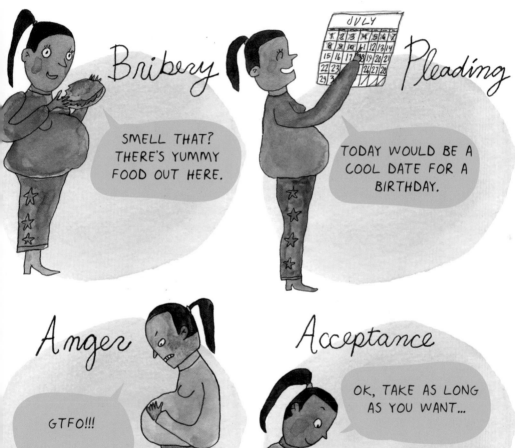

GROUP B STREP TEST

HAPPENS BETWEEN 36-37 WEEKS

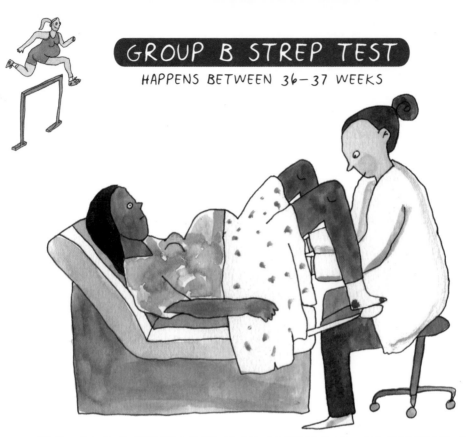

THE GROUP B STREP TEST IS TO SCREEN FOR GBS BACTERIA. THIS BACTERIA IS TOTALLY HARMLESS TO THE MOM, BUT VERY SERIOUS FOR A SMALL PERCENTAGE OF BABIES. SOURCES SAY THAT ABOUT ONE IN FOUR WOMEN WILL TEST POSITIVE FOR IT. YOUR DOCTOR WILL STICK A SWAB IN YOUR VAGINA AND BUTTHOLE. IF YOU TEST POSITIVE, THEY WILL HAVE YOU COME IN EARLIER IN YOUR LABOR TO GIVE YOU ANTIBIOTICS FOR THE BABY. IT'S DEFINITELY AN UNPLEASANT TEST, BUT AT LEAST IT'S QUICK.

TIP: IF YOU TEST POSITIVE, YOU CAN ALSO REQUEST TO BE RETESTED CLOSER TO THE DUE DATE IF YOU'D RATHER LABOR AT HOME LONGER.

YOU KEEP SEEING THINGS THAT REMIND YOU YOU'RE PREGNANT

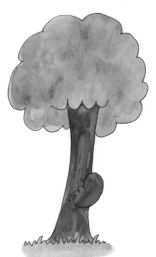

LUMPY TREE

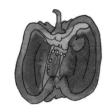

PEPPER WITH THE BABY PEPPER INSIDE

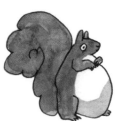

FAT SQUIRREL

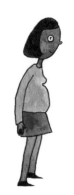

OTHER PREGNANT LADIES

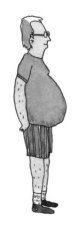

MAN WITH A GUT

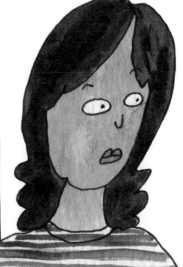

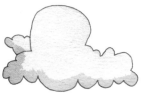

BULGING PURSE

EXPECTANT CLOUD

131

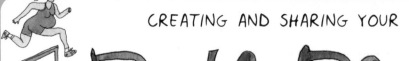

CREATING AND SHARING YOUR

Birth Plan

A BIRTH PLAN IS A GUIDELINE OF WHAT YOU WANT FOR YOUR BABY'S BIRTH. OF COURSE THEY ARE TOTALLY OPTIONAL. BELOW ARE SOME PROS AND CONS FOR CREATING ONE.

ADVANTAGES

☐ IF YOU THINK THROUGH YOUR OPTIONS BEFOREHAND (VIA BIRTH PLAN), IT CAN HELP YOU MAKE MORE INFORMED DECISIONS WHILE YOU ARE IN THE MOMENT OF GIVING BIRTH.

☐ IT MAY HELP YOU MENTALLY PREPARE FOR LABOR AND BIRTH.

☐ IT MAY HELP YOU FEEL MORE IN CONTROL.

☐ IT CAN BE A GOOD TOOL TO COMMUNICATE WITH MEDICAL PROFESSIONALS ABOUT YOUR BIRTH WISHES.

DISADVANTAGES

☐ IT TAKES TIME.

☐ IT MAY MAKE YOU THINK THROUGH SOME POTENTIALLY SCARY SITUATIONS.

☐ LABOR AND BIRTH MIGHT NOT GO THE WAY YOU PLANNED. (THIS IS ALMOST A GUARANTEE, TEE HEE HEE!)

IF YOU CREATE A BIRTH PLAN YOU'LL WANT TO SHARE IT WITH YOUR MEDICAL TEAM. WHAT FOLLOWS IS A LIST TO GET YOU STARTED ON YOUR BIRTH PLAN IF YOU CHOOSE TO CREATE ONE.

☐ WHAT HOPES DO YOU HAVE FOR THIS BIRTH?
VAGINAL BIRTH, NONTRAUMATIC BIRTH, HEALTHY BABY, HEALTHY MOMMY,_____

☐ WHAT FEARS DO YOU HAVE FOR THIS BIRTH?
PAIN, TRAUMATIC BIRTH, DEATH,_____

☐ WHAT IS YOUR DESIRED DELIVERY METHOD?
VBAC, C-SECTION, VAGINAL, WATER,_____

☐ WHO WOULD YOU LIKE IN THE ROOM?
PARTNER, MOM, DOULA,_____

☐ WHAT SORT OF VIBE DO YOU WANT FOR YOUR LABORING?
CALM, CHEERFUL, ROMANTIC,_____

☐ WHAT SORT OF VIBE DO YOU WANT FOR PUSHING?
HIGH ENERGY, TECHNO MUSIC, CALM, HEAVY METAL,_____

☐ WHAT DO YOU PLAN TO BRING TO HELP WITH THESE VIBES?
PLAYLIST/SPEAKERS, LOW LIGHTS, OWN CLOTHES,_____

☐ HOW YOU'D LIKE TO LABOR FIRST STAGE:
WALKING AROUND, IN THE SHOWER, WITH PEANUT BALL,_____

☐ WHAT YOU'D RATHER NOT HAVE DONE:
URINARY CATHETER, AN IV, EPISIOTOMY,_____

☐ WHAT TYPE OF LABOR AUGMENTATION YOU'D PREFER:
BREAK WATER, PITOCIN, BALLOON,_____

☐ WHAT TYPE OF PAIN RELIEF YOU'D LIKE TO USE:
EPIDURAL, MASSAGE, HYPNOSIS, YOU'LL DECIDE THAT DAY,
(FOR MORE OPTIONS SEE PAGES 140—143),_____

☐ WHAT POSITION YOU'D LIKE TO DELIVER IN:
ON BACK, IN TUB, SQUATTING,_____

☐ WHAT YOU'D PREFER FOR DELIVERY:
PUSH YOURSELF, HAVE THEM DIRECT YOUR PUSHING, AVOID
VACUUM, USE A MIRROR,_____

☐ AFTER DELIVERY:
YOU WANT PARTNER TO CUT CORD, YOU WANT TO CUT CORD, YOU
WANT TO SEE PLACENTA (RECOMMENDED!),_____

☐ IF A C—SECTION IS NEEDED, WHAT YOU WOULD LIKE:
SECOND OPINION, TO HAVE THE SURGERY EXPLAINED AS IT
HAPPENS, TO HAVE THE SCREEN LOWERED SO YOU CAN WATCH
THE BABY COME OUT,_____

☐ AFTER BIRTH YOU WOULD LIKE:
NO VISITORS FOR THE FIRST 24 HOURS, NO
VISITORS FOR THE FIRST 12 HOURS, ONLY
IMMEDIATE FAMILY,_____

☐ YOU WOULD LIKE THE FOLLOWING
PEOPLE NOT ALLOWED IN:

_____

☐ ANYTHING ELSE YOU WANT FOR IT?

_____

_____

PERINEAL MASSAGE
PREVENTATIVE CARE

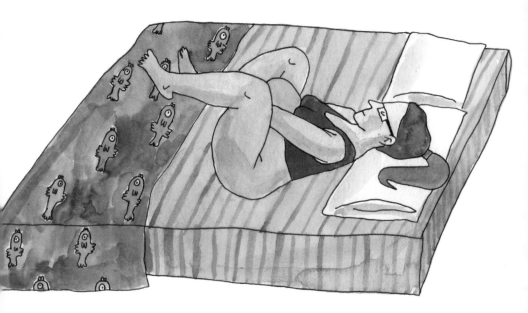

TOWARDS THE END OF PREGNANCY, WOMEN CAN START TO DO
PERINEAL MASSAGES. REALLY THESE ARE FANCY WORDS FOR HELPING
YOUR VAGINA GET FLEXIBLE FOR BIRTH. BASICALLY YOU STICK SOME
FINGERS IN AND STRETCH IT.* IT HAS BEEN SHOWN THAT REGULAR
PERINEAL MASSAGES IN THE LATER STAGES OF PREGNANCY CAN HELP
REDUCE TEARS, ESPECIALLY IN FIRST-TIME MOMS. MAYBE CALL IT
"YOGA FOR YOUR YONI."

*PLEASE GOOGLE ACTUAL DIRECTIONS FROM REPUTABLE SOURCE.

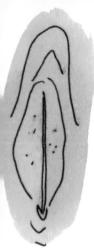

VAGINAL TEARS
A QUICK SUMMARY

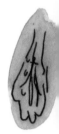

THE VAGINA IS AMAZING. IT CAN STRETCH TO THREE
TIMES ITS SIZE TO PUSH OUT AN ENTIRE BABY.
HOWEVER, THIS IDEA CAN BE STRESSFUL TO THINK
ABOUT PRIOR TO LABOR. WHAT IF IT TEARS?

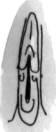

FIRST DEGREE: MOST COMMON TEAR. SMALL, ON
SKIN ONLY, HEALS QUICKLY. STILL HURTS LIKE A
BITCH.

SECOND DEGREE: AFFECTS MUSCLE, NEEDS STITCHES.

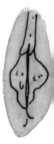

THIRD OR FOURTH DEGREE: MUCH LESS COMMON
(3.5%). MORE LIKELY TO HAPPEN WHEN USING A
VACUUM OR FORCEPS TO ASSIST DELIVERY, IF THE BABY
IS BIGGER, OR THE BABY IS BACK TO BACK WITH MOM.

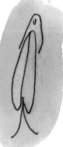
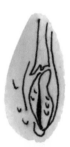
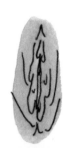
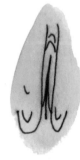

JUST NOT THINKING ABOUT IT

MAYBE YOU DON'T WANT TO THINK ABOUT A BIRTH PLAN, AND YOU DON'T WANT TO THINK ABOUT WHAT MIGHT HAPPEN TO YOUR VAGINA. AND THAT'S OK. EVEN IF EVERYONE KEEPS ASKING IF YOU'RE READY, AND YOU WONDER WHAT "BEING READY" WOULD EVEN ENTAIL. YOU HAVEN'T BEEN THINKING ABOUT IT TOO MUCH. IT FEELS LIKE IT'S JUST GOING TO HAPPEN, AND THERE'S SO MUCH UNKNOWN THAT YOU'LL DRIVE YOURSELF CRAZY IF YOU KEEP THINKING ABOUT IT, SO YOU STOP. YOU JUST TRY TO RELAX, AND TRY TO SLEEP, AND YOU WAIT.

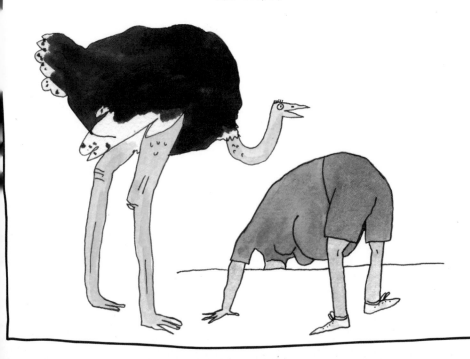

At Nine Months

POOP BEING CREATED

LUNGS WORKING

HANDS ABLE TO GRASP

WEEKS 37–42

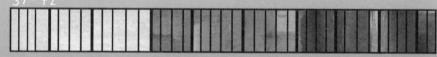

THE FINAL MONTH! ANY DAY NOW, IT'S GOING TO HAPPEN.

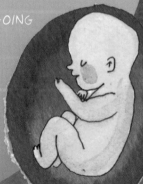

AVERAGE SIZE AT END OF 40 WEEKS: 20.16 IN (51.2 CM)

TURNING THE BREECH BABY
(EXTERNAL CEPHALIC VERSION)

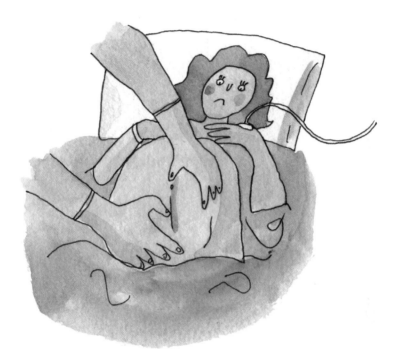

AT 37 WEEKS YOUR BABY IS STILL BREECH. YOUR DOCTOR OFFERS TO TRY ECV TO TURN THE BABY MANUALLY. YOU DECIDE TO TRY IT EVEN THOUGH YOU READ MIXED REVIEWS ONLINE. YOU AREN'T ALLOWED TO EAT FOR EIGHT HOURS BEFORE AND YOU ARE VERY NERVOUS. IT HURTS—A LOT. YOUR BABY FLIPS! HOWEVER, BY THE NEXT TIME YOU GO IN, HE HAS FLIPPED BACK. YOU SCHEDULE A C-SECTION HAPPILY, KNOWING YOU TRIED EVERYTHING!

PAIN RELIEF DURING LABOR

SOME PEOPLE TALK ABOUT THEIR WONDERFUL, ORGASMIC LABOR, AND YOU MAY WONDER, "WILL THAT BE ME?" MAYBE. BUT IT'S ALWAYS A GOOD IDEA TO KNOW ABOUT YOUR PAIN MANAGEMENT OPTIONS BEFORE YOU ARE IN THE MOMENT—ESPECIALLY IF THAT MOMENT IS SOMETHING YOU'VE NEVER DONE BEFORE, LIKE BRINGING A HUMAN INTO THE WORLD.

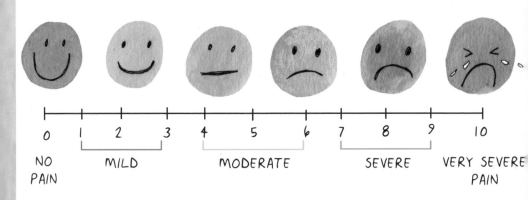

FOR MANY, LABOR STARTS OFF IN THE MILD-TO-MODERATE ZONE AND THEN JUMPS TO VERY SEVERE (SOMETIMES AFTER THE WATER BREAKS OR IS BROKEN).

THE TYPES OF PAIN MEDICATION THAT WILL BE AVAILABLE TO YOU WILL DEPEND ON WHAT'S AVAILABLE AT YOUR BIRTHING LOCATION. IN THE NEXT FEW PAGES YOU'LL FIND SHORT SUMMARIES OF SOME COMMON PAIN RELIEF OPTIONS.

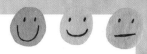

MOVEMENT/POSITIONS

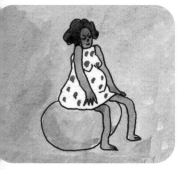

IF YOU'RE ABLE, IT CAN HELP TO MOVE AROUND TO DIFFERENT POSITIONS WHILE IN LABOR. MANY HOSPITALS OFFER YOGA BALLS OR BARS FOR THIS PURPOSE.

WATER

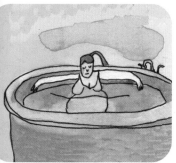

ALWAYS A SOOTHING PRESENCE, A TUB WITH JETS OR EVEN A WARM SHOWER CAN HELP YOU GET THROUGH CONTRACTIONS.

MUSIC

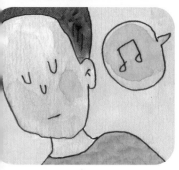

ESPECIALLY USEFUL DURING THE EARLY STAGES OF LABOR OR THE LATER STAGES FOR PUSHING, MUSIC CAN HELP YOU STAY IN THE ZONE.

DISTRACTION

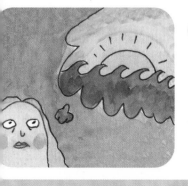

THE MIND IS A POWERFUL TOOL FOR DEALING WITH PAIN. IT CAN HELP TO PICTURE YOURSELF SOMEWHERE ELSE OR FOCUS ON A PARTICULAR THING IN THE ROOM.

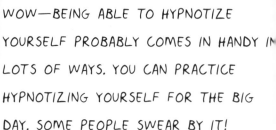

HYPNOBIRTHING

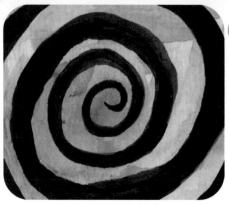

WOW—BEING ABLE TO HYPNOTIZE YOURSELF PROBABLY COMES IN HANDY IN LOTS OF WAYS. YOU CAN PRACTICE HYPNOTIZING YOURSELF FOR THE BIG DAY. SOME PEOPLE SWEAR BY IT!

BREATHING

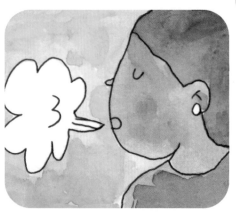

LEARNING HOW TO USE BREATH AS A TOOL TO RELIEVE PAIN AND STRESS IS A VALUABLE LIFE SKILL AND WONDER-FUL TECHNIQUE FOR CHILDBIRTH. LIKE HYPNOBIRTHING, IT'S DEFINITELY SOMETHING YOU WOULD HAVE TO PRACTICE AHEAD OF TIME.

MASSAGE

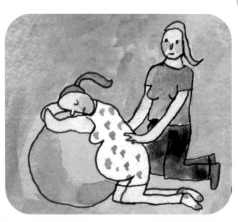

SOMEONE APPLYING PRESSURE ON DIFFERENT PARTS OF YOUR BODY CAN CERTAINLY HELP YOU TOLERATE THE PAIN OF LABOR. DOULAS NORMALLY KNOW WHAT TO DO AND CAN ALSO TEACH YOUR PARTNER. BE VOCAL ABOUT WHAT FEELS GOOD.

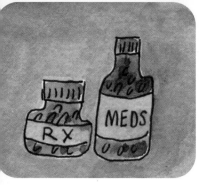

NARCOTICS

A GREAT OPTION IF YOU DON'T WANT OR CAN'T HAVE AN EPIDURAL BUT YOU WANT SOME BIG-TIME PAIN MANAGEMENT HELP.

LAUGHING GAS

LESS COMMON IN THE US, GAS CAN BE A GREAT TOOL TO USE IN LABOR TO DISASSOCIATE FROM THE PAIN. IT'S A GOOD OPTION TO TRY IF YOU WANT TO BE ABLE TO MOVE AROUND.

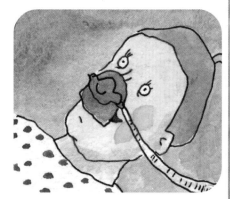

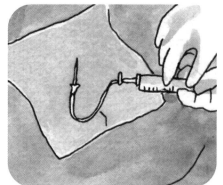

EPIDURAL

THE BIG MAMA OF PAIN RELIEF. IT'S OK AND NORMAL IF YOU FEEL SCARED OF THIS. IT IS LITERALLY A NEEDLE GOING IN YOUR SPINE. MANY WOMEN KNOW THAT THEY WANT THIS, OTHERS AREN'T DECIDED, AND STILL OTHERS WOULD RATHER SKIP IT. THERE ARE A LOT OF OPINIONS OUT THERE, BUT REALLY ONLY YOU KNOW WHAT'S RIGHT FOR YOU.

NEEDING TO BE HORIZONTAL

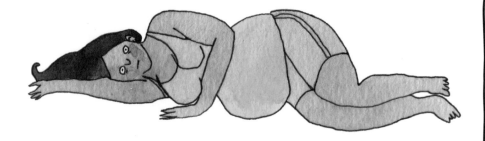

YOUR PREGNANCY HASN'T BEEN EASY. YOU HAVE GESTATIONAL DIABETES AND WORK HAS BEEN REALLY STRESSFUL. BY THE TIME YOU GET TO YOUR NINTH MONTH YOU HAVE THIS CONSTANT NEED TO BE HORIZONTAL. IT'S TOUGH STAYING UP PAST 8 PM.

SOMETIMES WHEN YOU COMPLAIN ABOUT HOW TIRED YOU ARE TO YOUR FRIENDS, THEY EMPATHIZE WITH YOU BY SAYING "I ALSO HAVEN'T MOVED FROM THE COUCH IN HOURS, AND I'M NOT EVEN PREGNANT." IT BRINGS YOU COMFORT TO KNOW THAT OTHERS ARE ALSO EXHAUSTED AND THEY AREN'T EVEN MAKING A BABY!

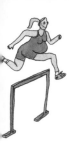

Third Trimester

DOCTOR VISITS

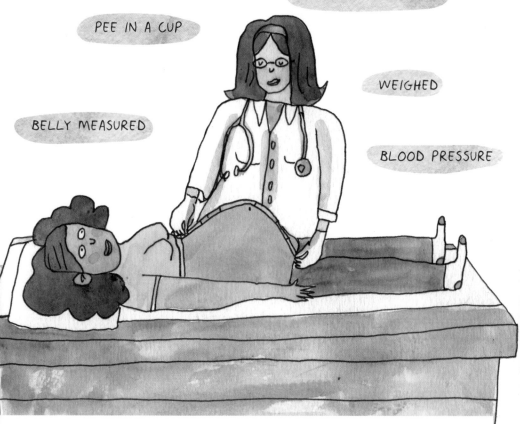

BABY'S HEARTBEAT

PEE IN A CUP

WEIGHED

BELLY MEASURED

BLOOD PRESSURE

BY THE THIRD TRIMESTER YOU'LL BE SEEING YOUR DOCTOR A LOT (EVERY WEEK OR EVERY OTHER WEEK). THE VISITS LIKELY WON'T TAKE LONG, BUT IT'S A GOOD CHANCE TO TALK TO YOUR DOCTOR ABOUT ANY QUESTIONS OR CONCERNS YOU MAY HAVE. ALONG WITH THE ABOVE, YOU'LL LIKELY GET A FLU SHOT AND TDAP VACCINE, WHICH WILL PASS ANTIBODIES TO YOUR BABY IN THE FIRST MONTHS OF LIFE.

PREGNANCY PHOTO SHOOT

ONE WAY TO CELEBRATE THE BIG BUMP IS TO DO A PHOTO SHOOT.

THERE ARE MANY WAYS TO DO IT:

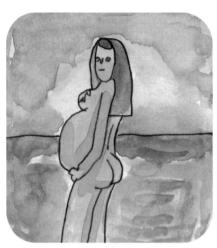

NAKED WITH GREEN SCREEN

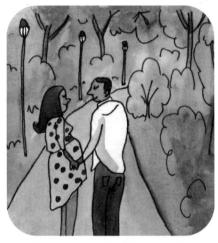

FULLY CLOTHED CLASSY
WOODS SHOOT

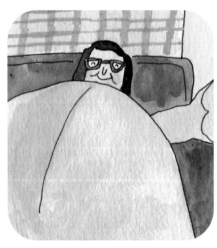

FUNNY SELFIES

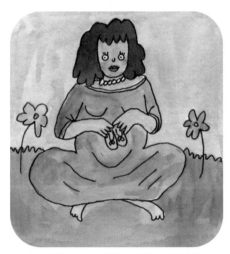

ANGELIC WITH BABY PROPS

OR NOT AT ALL!

FUN WITH THE BELLY

BESIDES TAKING PHOTOS, HAVING A BIG BELLY IS AN OPPORTUNITY TO HAVE SOME FUN. SOME EXAMPLES BELOW:

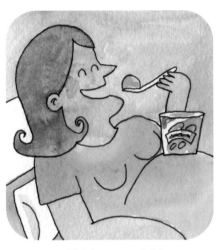

ICE CREAM HOLDER

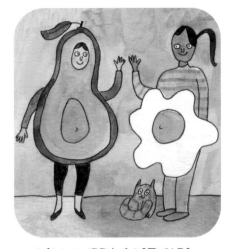

HALLOWEEN COSTUMES

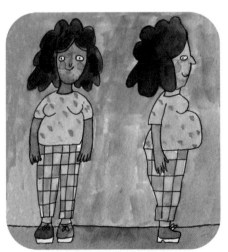

COMPARING FRONT TO PROFILE VIEWS

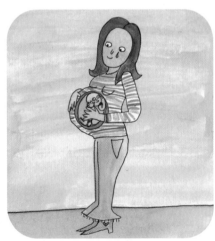

PLAYING EXISTENTIAL MIND GAMES ABOUT HOW YOU ARE NEVER ALONE

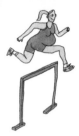

THERE COMES A MOMENT IN EVERY PREGNANCY WHEN...

I CAN'T SEE MY VAGINA.

SOME FIND IT LIBERATING, SOME ASK THEIR PARTNERS TO HELP TRIM, BUT WE CAN ALL ADMIT IT'S PRETTY IRONIC THAT YOU ARE LITERALLY GROWING A BABY SO BIG THAT IT'S IMPEDED YOUR VIEW OF THE HOLE IT'S MEANT TO COME OUT OF.

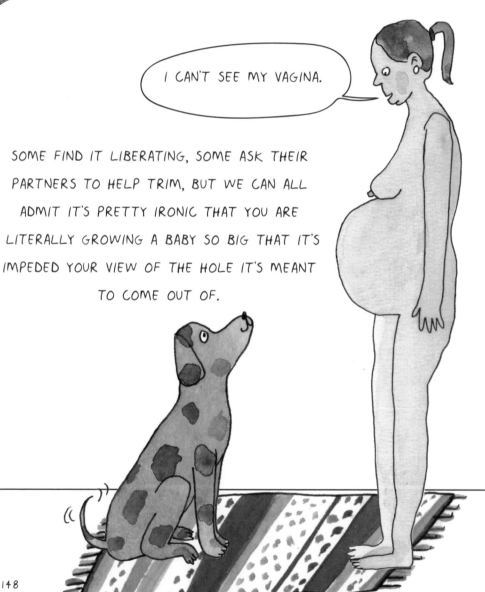

CLEANING THE ENTIRE HOUSE

THERE REALLY DOES SEEM TO BE SOMETHING ABOUT BEING IN THE LATER STAGES OF PREGNANCY THAT MAKES ONE FEEL LIKE CLEANING—A LOT. CLEANING IS A NESTING INSTINCT THAT CAN HAPPEN AT ANY POINT DURING PREGNANCY, OR NOT AT ALL, OR EVEN WHEN NOT PREGNANT. MANY A TALE IS TOLD OF WOMEN IN THE THIRD TRIMESTER WHO SPEND THE DAY CLEANING, HARD, AND FIND THAT THEY GO INTO LABOR SOON AFTER. EVEN IF THAT DOESN'T HAPPEN, WORST—CASE SCENARIO: A CLEAN HOUSE.

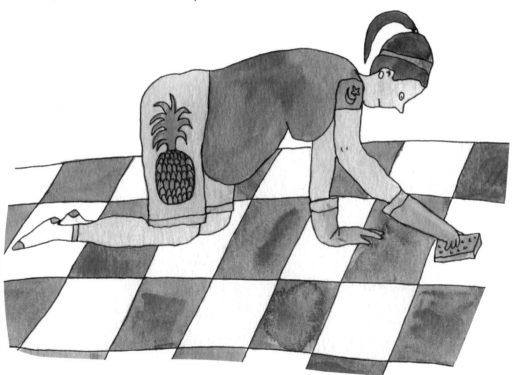

Mini Contractions

LIKELY BY THE THIRD TRIMESTER YOU'LL HAVE STARTED TO EXPERIENCE "BRAXTON HICKS." THE NAME IS JUST BASED ON SOME OLD BRITISH DOCTOR WHO "DISCOVERED" THEM, LIKE HOW COLUMBUS DISCOVERED AMERICA. WE SHOULD ALL START CALLING THEM MINI CONTRACTIONS BECAUSE THAT'S BASICALLY WHAT THEY ARE.

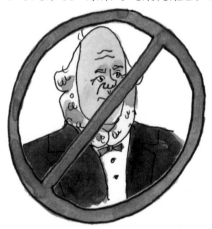

MINI CONTRACTIONS CAN FEEL LIKE YOU'RE DOING A CRUNCH, PERIOD CRAMPS, INTENSE PAIN IN THE HIPS OR BACK, A SQUEEZING FEELING, OR SOMETHING ELSE!

NO ONE SEEMS TO TALK ABOUT HOW COMMON IT IS TO HAVE THESE MINI CONTRACTIONS START AND STOP, SOMETIMES FOR WEEKS AND MONTHS LEADING UP TO LABOR. MISTAKING THESE MINI CONTRACTIONS FOR ACTUAL LABOR IS TOTALLY NORMAL, AND AT TIMES CAN MAKE YOU FEEL LIKE...

...THE PREGNANT WOMAN WHO CRIED...

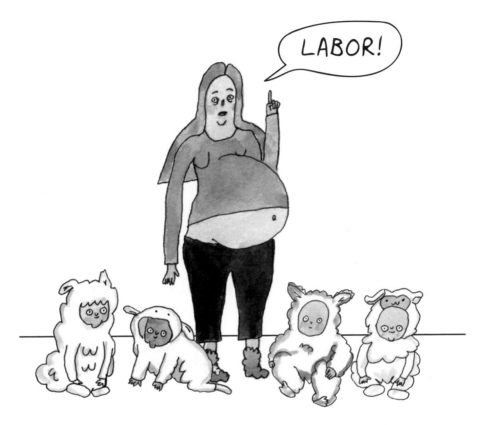

YOU MAY CONTINUE HAVING A BUNCH OF FALSE ALARMS UP UNTIL THE BIG DAY. AGAIN, TOTALLY NORMAL. YOUR BODY IS PREPPING.

FOR MOST WOMEN, THE ONLY WAY TO SPOT THAT IT'S "REAL LABOR" IS WHEN CONTRACTIONS COME AT SHORT INTERVALS (3 TO 5 MINUTES APART), LAST A CERTAIN AMOUNT OF TIME (ONE MINUTE), AND DO SO FOR AN HOUR. TIME TO HEAD TO THE HOSPITAL IF SO!

INDUCING LABOR?

YOU FEEL LIKE A CAR TRYING TO START UP WHEN YOU GET MINI CONTRACTIONS THAT COME AND GO.

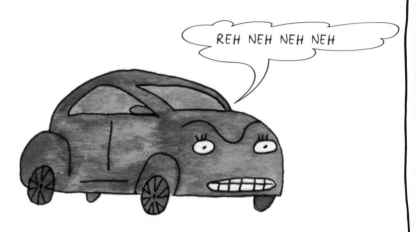

REH NEH NEH NEH

YOU GO ON A WALK AND YOU FEEL CONTRACTIONS IN A PATTERN AND ARE PRETTY SURE THIS IS IT!

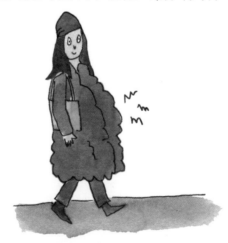

BUT THEN THEY GO AWAY, LIKE THEY HAVE BEEN FOR THE LAST COUPLE WEEKS. WHEN YOU GET HOME, DISAPPOINTED, YOUR HUSBAND SAYS:

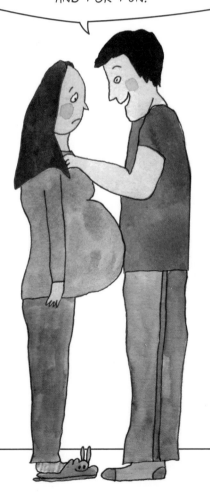

MAYBE WE SHOULD TRY SEX TO HELP INDUCE... AND FOR FUN!

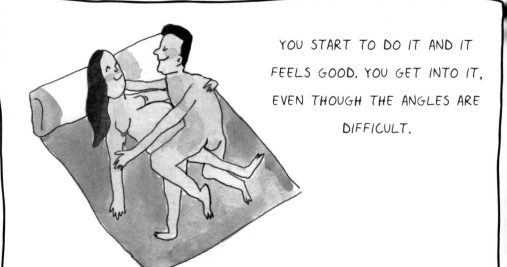

YOU START TO DO IT AND IT FEELS GOOD. YOU GET INTO IT, EVEN THOUGH THE ANGLES ARE DIFFICULT.

ALL OF A SUDDEN, HE STOPS AND POINTS OUT A GIANT WET SPOT ON THE BED.

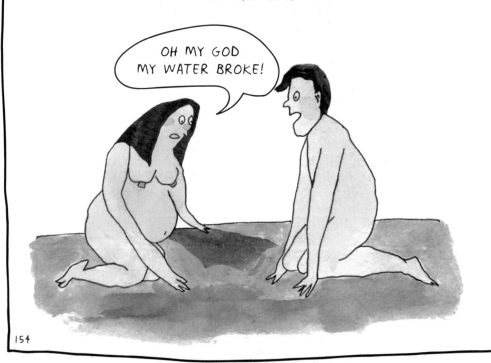

OH MY GOD MY WATER BROKE!

BUT THEN YOU REALIZE THAT IT WASN'T YOUR WATER BREAKING, IT
WAS ACTUALLY A WATER BOTTLE THAT WAS IN THE BED AND HAD
SPILLED. YOU LAUGH YOUR BUTT OFF. EVEN THOUGH THE SEX DIDN'T
HELP GET LABOR STARTED, IT DID CHEER YOU UP, AND THAT'S REALLY
ALL THAT MATTERS.

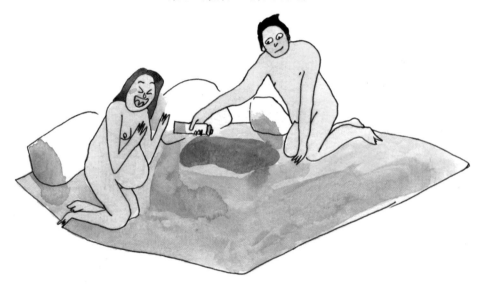

NOTE ON WATER BREAKING: IF YOUR WATER BREAKS OR YOU THINK IT
BROKE (SOMETIMES IT'S NOT A BIG SPLASH BUT A SMALL LEAK) THEN
YOU SHOULD MAKE NOTE OF THE TIME YOU THINK IT HAPPENED AND
CALL YOUR HEALTH CARE PROVIDER TO DISCUSS NEXT STEPS.

YOUR DUE DATE COMES AND GOES...

SO YOU BASICALLY TRY EVERY SUGGESTED INDUCTION METHOD OUT THERE. YOU DON'T REALLY BELIEVE THEY WORK BUT AT THIS POINT YOU'LL TRY ANYTHING!

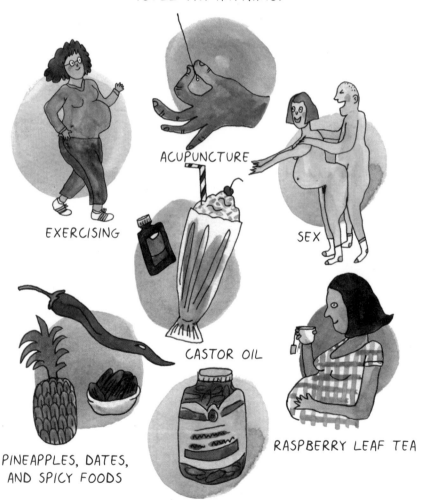

EXERCISING

ACUPUNCTURE

SEX

CASTOR OIL

PINEAPPLES, DATES, AND SPICY FOODS

RASPBERRY LEAF TEA

Third Trimester

BY THE END OF THE THIRD TRIMESTER YOU WILL LIKELY HAVE
ACCOMPLISHED THE FOLLOWING:

POTENTIAL TO-DOS

TOUR THE HOSPITAL OR BIRTHING CENTER. IF PLANNING A
HOME BIRTH, THEN PREPARE FOR THAT AT HOME

CREATE AND SHARE YOUR BIRTH PLAN IF YOU WANTED ONE

PACK A BAG

START PERINEAL MASSAGES IF YOU PLANNED TO DO THEM

TAKE A BABY 101 CLASS—WITH YOUR COPARENT, SO THEY
LEARN HOW TO SWADDLE, TOO. (THERE ARE ALSO SOME
FREE CLASSES ONLINE!)

PREP SOME FREEZER MEALS AND ONE-HANDED SNACKS

LINE UP HELP FOR WHEN THE BABY COMES

Labor & Birth

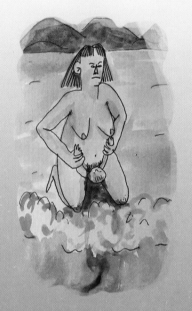

IT'S FINALLY
HAPPENING

The Unknown

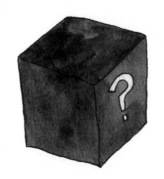

THE ONLY THING YOU KNOW FOR SURE IS THAT YOU'RE HOPING TO GET A BABY AT THE END OF THIS PROCESS. MOST EVERYTHING ELSE—HOW IT WILL HAPPEN, WHEN IT WILL HAPPEN, HOW MUCH IT WILL HURT—IS A MYSTERY. UNLESS OF COURSE YOU ARE HAVING A SCHEDULED C-SECTION, THEN YOU KNOW A LITTLE MORE.

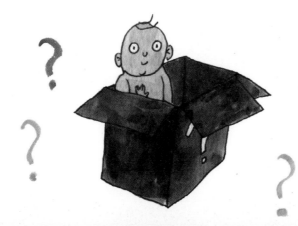

CERVIX: 1–3 CENTIMETERS DILATED

AS PREVIOUSLY MENTIONED, THE FIRST STAGES OF LABOR CAN FEEL
LIKE NOTHING OR LIKE DIFFERENT TYPES OF MILD TO MODERATE
PAIN. THE GOOD NEWS IS, YOU REALLY DON'T NEED TO DO MUCH
EXCEPT PERHAPS REST AT THIS STAGE. MOST WOMEN ARE ONLY SUR
IT'S TIME WHEN THE PAIN GETS STRONGER AND THE CONTRACTIONS
COME AT QUICKER INTERVALS.

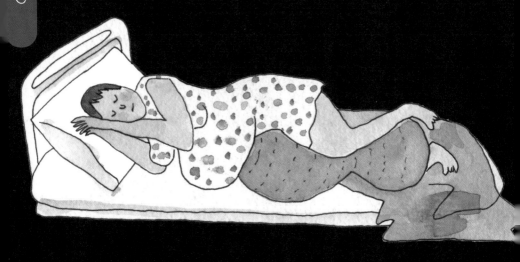

THE HORMONE OXYTOCIN IS RESPONSIBLE FOR THE CONTRACTIONS.
OFTEN CALLED THE "LOVE HORMONE," WE ALSO FEEL IT DURING
INTIMATE BONDING TIMES LIKE SEX AND BREASTFEEDING.

AFTER TRANSITIONING (4–5 CM) YOU ARE OFFICIALLY IN ACTIVE LABOR. THIS IS WHEN THINGS REALLY GET REAL (READ: PAINFUL). IT'S TIME FOR SOME SERIOUS PAIN MANAGEMENT, FOR MOST PEOPLE.

CERVIX: 5.5–8 CENTIMETERS DILATED

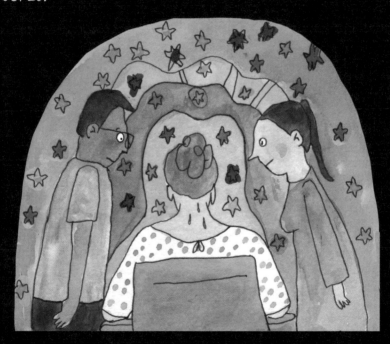

SUPPOSEDLY, STAYING RELAXED AND CONFIDENT WILL HELP THE CONTRACTIONS CONTINUE TO BUILD, WHILE BECOMING STRESSED CAN LEAD TO LESS OXYTOCIN AND POTENTIALLY SLOW DOWN LABOR. THE GENERAL ADVICE HERE IS TO RELAX—MUCH EASIER SAID THAN DONE.

CONTRACTIONS: 2-4 MINUTES APART

IF YOU GET AN EPIDURAL, ACTIVE LABOR MAY LOOK LIKE YOU LYING IN THE HOSPITAL BED TRYING TO SLEEP, BUT LABORING THIS WAY CAN STILL BE VERY, VERY HARD. YOUR BODY IS DOING A LOT OF WORK RIGHT NOW—AND SO ARE YOU.

CERVIX: 5.5-8 CENTIMETERS DILATED

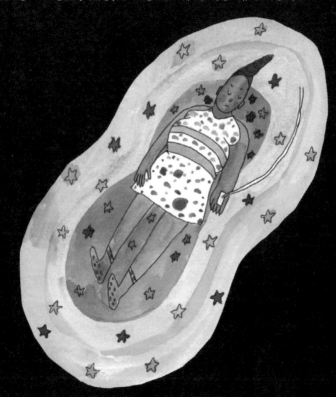

SOMETIMES REFERRED TO AS THE "MOTHERING HORMONE," PROLACTIN WILL GRADUALLY INCREASE IN YOUR BODY UNTIL BIRTH. IT ALSO HELPS WITH BREASTFEEDING.

PUSHING

CONTRACTIONS: 2 – 3 MINUTES APART

FINALLY, IT'S TIME TO PUSH. YOUR DOCTOR MAY TELL YOU TO MAKE LIKE YOU'RE TAKING A POOP (AND YOU WILL LIKELY POOP AT SOME POINT—BUT SERIOUSLY DON'T STRESS OUT ABOUT IT, IT'LL BE THE LAST THING ON YOUR MIND BY THIS POINT). SOME PEOPLE CHOOSE TO USE A MIRROR TO HELP THEM SEE THEIR EFFORTS.

CERVIX: 10 CENTIMETERS DILATED

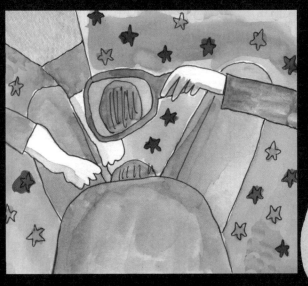

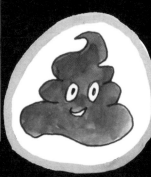

ADRENALINE WILL PROBABLY KICK IN FOR PUSHING IF IT HASN'T ALREADY. MANY WOMEN FEEL A SURGE OF ENERGY AT THIS POINT TO HELP THEM FINISH THE JOB.

PUSHING: A TIP

IT CAN BE VERY DIFFICULT TO IMAGINE THE MOMENT OF ACTUALLY PUSHING AND HOW YOU'LL DO IT. YOU CAN EITHER DECIDE WHEN TO PUSH OR YOUR DOCTOR OR MIDWIFE WILL COUNT BACKWARDS WHILE YOU EXHALE AND PUSH. IT'S IMPORTANT TO DO ONE LONG PUSH INSTEAD OF A BUNCH OF SMALL PUSHES DURING THOSE SECONDS. THIS IS THE TIME TO GIVE IT YOUR ALL.

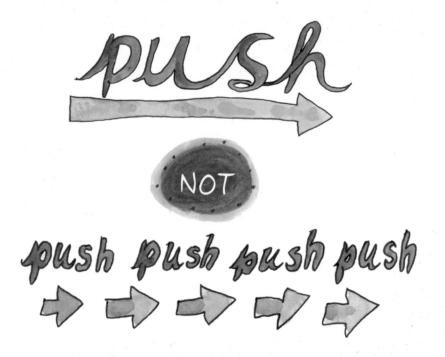

SLOW OR FAST, THERE'S NO ONE RIGHT WAY, AND GOING AT YOUR OWN PACE MAY HELP YOU TEAR LESS, SINCE YOU'RE GIVING YOUR VAGINA TIME TO STRETCH OUT. DO WHAT FEELS RIGHT TO YOU.

Induction

20-40% OF LABORS ARE NOW INDUCED. IT MIGHT FEEL LIKE THE BELOW—ALL STRAPPED IN AND READY TO GO.

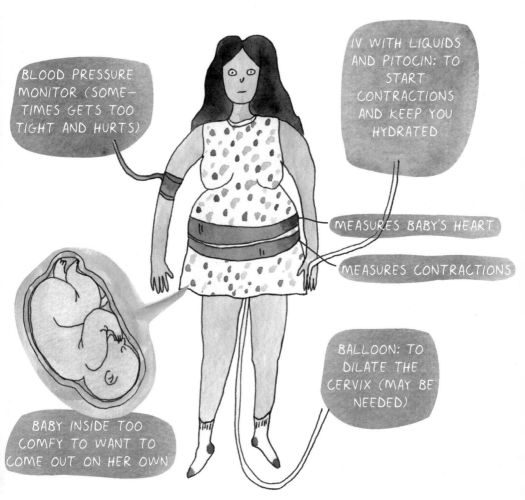

BLOOD PRESSURE MONITOR (SOME-TIMES GETS TOO TIGHT AND HURTS)

IV WITH LIQUIDS AND PITOCIN: TO START CONTRACTIONS AND KEEP YOU HYDRATED

MEASURES BABY'S HEART

MEASURES CONTRACTIONS

BALLOON: TO DILATE THE CERVIX (MAY BE NEEDED)

BABY INSIDE TOO COMFY TO WANT TO COME OUT ON HER OWN

REMEMBER: YOU CAN ALWAYS ASK QUESTIONS ABOUT WHAT IS BEING DONE AND WHY. IF YOU FEEL WEIRD ABOUT SOMETHING—ASK!

THE BIRTH PLAN

YOU SPEND A LOT OF TIME THINKING ABOUT HOW YOU WANT YOUR BIRTH TO GO. YOU DECIDE YOU WANT TO HAVE AS *LITTLE* MEDICAL INTERVENTION AS POSSIBLE AND WILL WAIT IT OUT TO SEE IF YOU WANT AN EPIDURAL OR NOT.

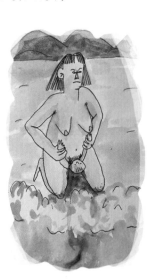

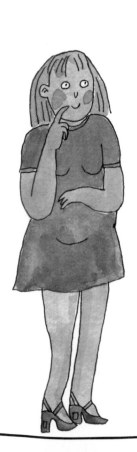

HOWEVER, AT 40 WEEKS YOU DECIDE TO SCHEDULE AN INDUCTION FOR THE FOLLOWING WEEK IN CASE YOU DON'T GO INTO LABOR BEFORE THEN. YOU DON'T, SO AT ALMOST 42 WEEKS YOU WAKE UP EARLY AND HEAD TO THE HOSPITAL.

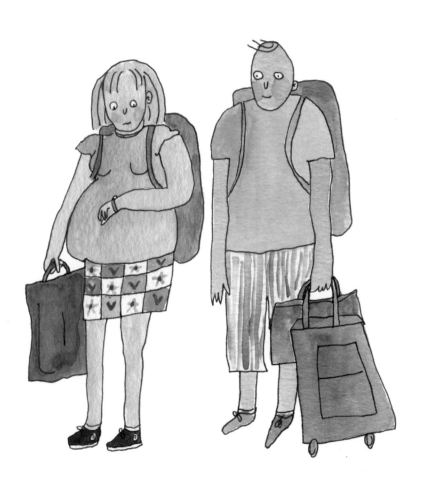

AT THE HOSPITAL YOU GET A BALLOON, PITOCIN, AN IV, YOUR WATER
BROKEN BY A DOCTOR, AND EVENTUALLY AN EPIDURAL. THE BIRTH
PLAN DID NOT GO AS EXPECTED. YOU HAD IMAGINED YOU'D HAVE AS
CLOSE TO A "NATURAL" BIRTH AS POSSIBLE, BUT THE OPPOSITE IS
TRUE—YOU GOT ALMOST ALL THE MEDICAL INTERVENTIONS YOU
COULD THINK OF.

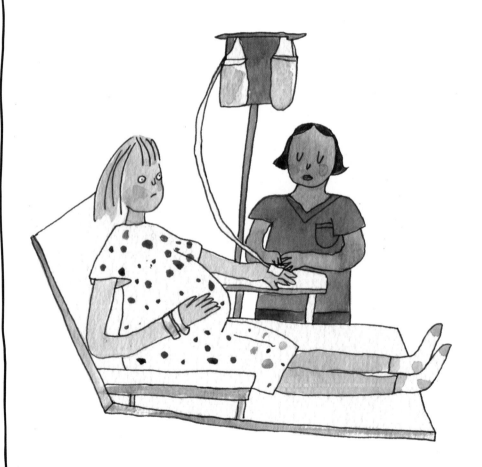

HOWEVER, IN THE END, THE FACT THAT THINGS DIDN'T GO AS PLANNED DOESN'T MATTER. WHAT YOU NOTICE IS THAT YOU AND YOUR BABY ARE BOTH HEALTHY, AND REALLY THAT WAS THE MOST IMPORTANT PART OF THE PLAN ALL ALONG.

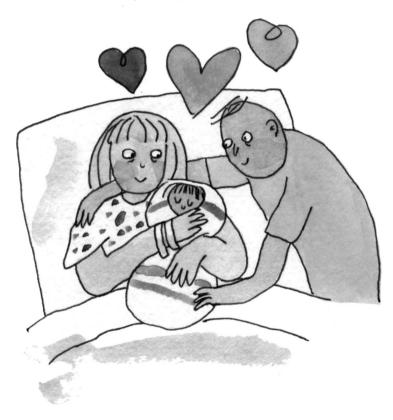

VAGINAL BIRTH

IN THE US, TWO OUT OF THREE WOMEN GIVE BIRTH VAGINALLY. IF MOM AND BABY ARE HEALTHY AND THERE ARE NO COMPLICATIONS, IT'S GENERALLY THE WAY TO GO. THANKFULLY, THERE IS ALWAYS THE OPTION OF A CAESAREAN IF THE NEED ARISES. PRAISE BE TO MODERN MEDICINE!

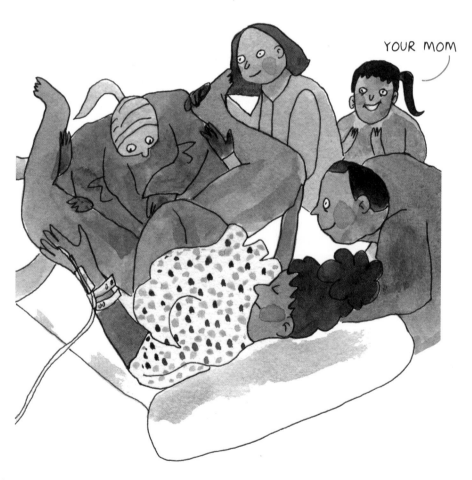

YOUR MOM

THE PEP TALK

ABOUT TEN HOURS INTO YOUR LABOR YOU FIND OUT THAT YOU'RE FULLY DILATED, HOWEVER THE BABY IS STILL REALLY HIGH UP. SO YOU ARE ADVISED TO WAIT TO PUSH. YOUR DOULA COMES OVER TO ASK HOW YOU'RE FEELING.

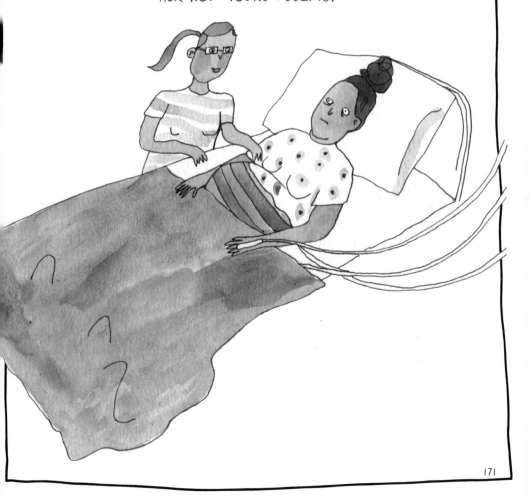

YOU TELL HER,

I'M SCARED. MY EPIDURAL IS WEARING OFF, AND I CAN SORT OF FEEL SOME OF THE CONTRACTIONS AGAIN. I WASN'T ABLE TO SLEEP, AND I DON'T FEEL GOOD. I'M FINALLY FACING THE FACT THAT I AM AFRAID OF HOW THE ACTUAL DELIVERY PART WILL GO.

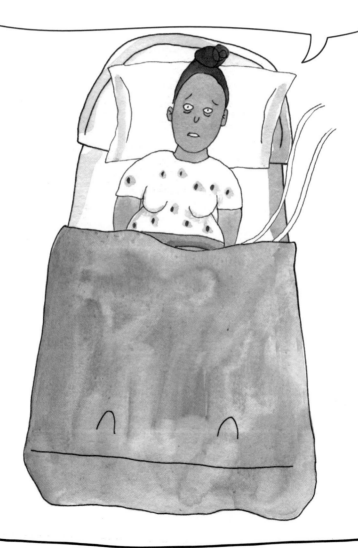

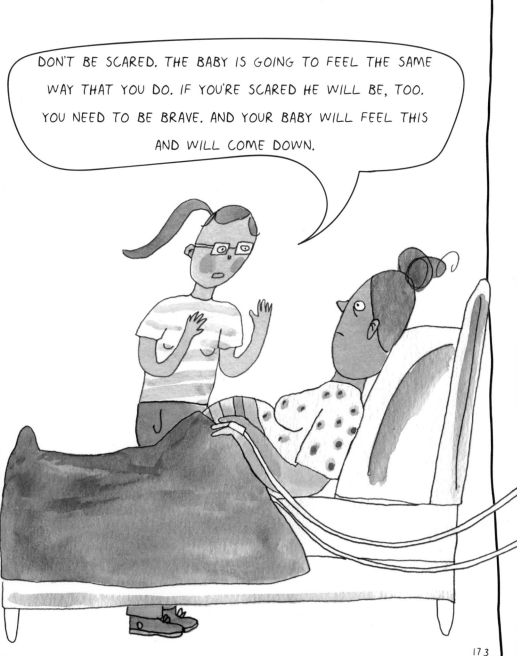

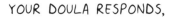

YOU TAKE IN WHAT SHE SAYS. YOU REALIZE SHE'S RIGHT. SO YOU SPEND THE NEXT HOUR PEP TALKING TO THE BABY, AND IN A WAY, YOURSELF.

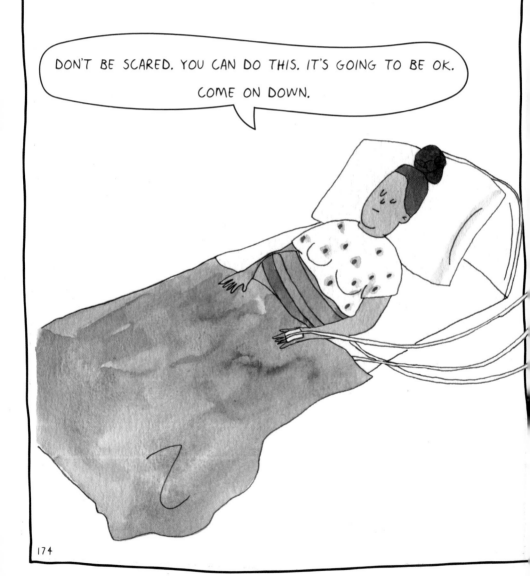

DON'T BE SCARED. YOU CAN DO THIS. IT'S GOING TO BE OK. COME ON DOWN.

AFTER ABOUT AN HOUR YOUR DOCTOR DOES ANOTHER CHECK. THE BABY HAS MOVED DOWN AND IT'S TIME TO PUSH! YOU ARE SHOCKED AND HAPPY THAT YOUR PEP TALK WORKED. YOU PUSH FOR AN HOUR AND BABY COMES OUT HEALTHY.

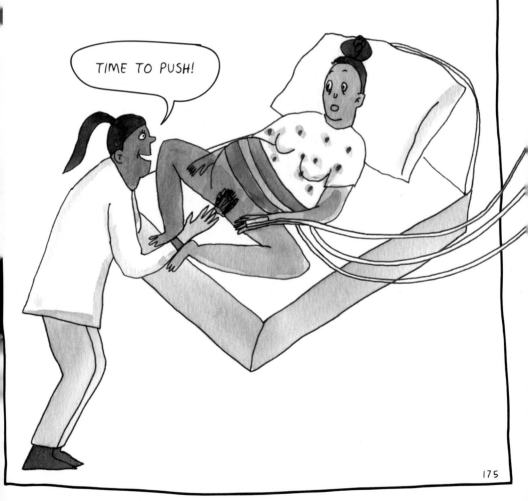

C-SECTION

THERE ARE MANY VARIED REASONS THAT ABOUT A THIRD OF WOMEN IN THE US HAVE A C-SECTION, INCLUDING:

- ☑ PROLONGED LABOR
- ☑ OBSTRUCTED LABOR
- ☑ BREECH BABY
- ☑ MULTIPLES
- ☑ HIGH BLOOD PRESSURE

- ☑ ISSUES WITH UMBILICAL CORD
- ☑ PROBLEMS WITH PLACENTA
- ☑ PREVIOUS C-SECTION BIRTH
- ☑ PREVIOUS TRAUMATIC BIRTH
- ☑ ELECTIVE FOR ANY OTHER REASON

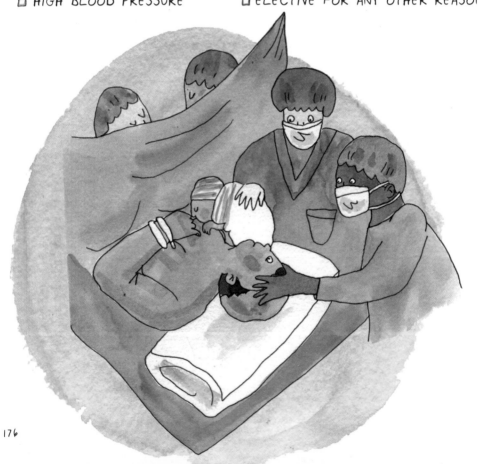

PLANNED C-SECTION

YOUR BABY WAS BREECH SO YOU SCHEDULED A C-SECTION. WHEN IT'S HAPPENING, YOU FEEL LOTS OF TUGGING AND PULLING, AND NO PAIN. AFTER, YOU WERE ASKED TO WAIT IN THE ROOM ALONE UNTIL YOU REGAINED FEELING IN YOUR LEGS, WHILE THE BABY AND YOUR PARTNER WENT SOMEWHERE ELSE.

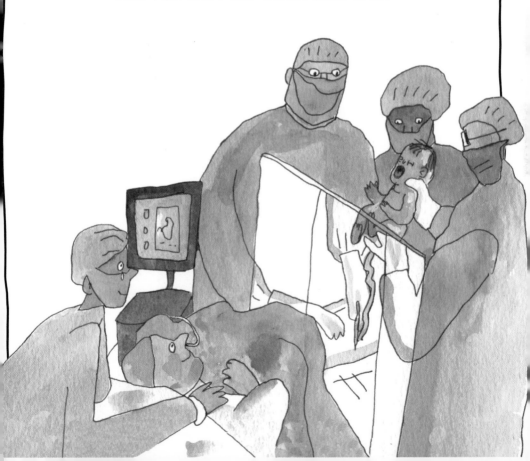

SOMETIMES, WHEN OTHERS DESCRIBE THEIR LABOR AND BABY'S BIRTH, YOU FEEL LEFT OUT, BECAUSE YOURS WAS SO DIFFERENT. HOWEVER, YOUR EXPERIENCE WAS AS REAL AS ANYONE ELSE'S. AND TO BE HONEST, SOME WOULD HAVE KILLED TO BE AT THE HOSPITAL AT 6 AM AND HAVE THE BABY OUT BY 9 AM LIKE YOU! AND AGAIN, THE MOST IMPORTANT THING IS THAT YOU ARE BOTH HEALTHY.

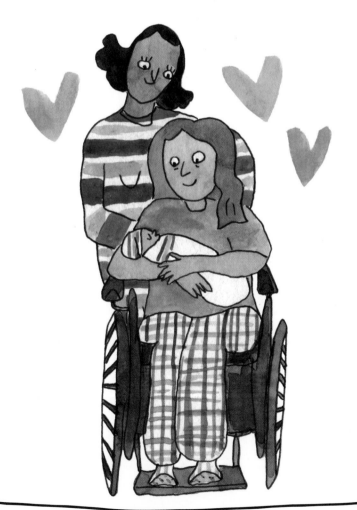

HE'S PERFECT!

HOWEVER IT HAPPENS, THE IMPORTANT THING IS THAT IT'S YOUR CHILD'S BIRTHDAY TODAY! HOPEFULLY DURING HIS BIRTH YOU FELT SUPPORTED AND HEARD WITH A CHEERING TEAM ON YOUR SIDE.

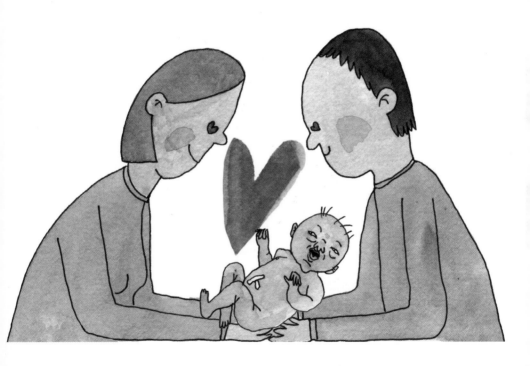

MOST NEWBORNS TRULY LOOK LIKE WRINKLED OLD GOBLINS, BUT OF COURSE, IN THE EYES OF EVERY NEW PARENT, THEIR BABY IS THE EXCEPTION.

Fourth Trimester

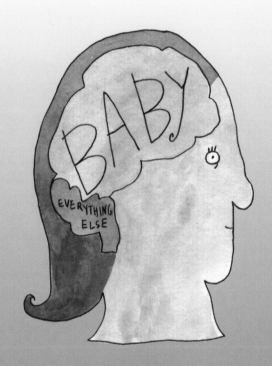

NEWBORN

BRAND SPANKING NEW!

BECOMING A MOM

ALL YOUR LIFE, YOU'VE HAD AN IDEA OF WHAT YOU THINK A MOM IS, FROM YOUR OWN MOM, FROM MOVIES, FROM SOCIETY. THEN, AFTER A LONG JOURNEY OF PREGNANCY AND GIVING BIRTH, YOU BECOME ONE. THE PAST NINE MONTHS YOU WEREN'T JUST CREATING A BABY, YOU WERE ALSO CREATING A MOTHER, AND POTENTIALLY ANOTHER PARENT. IT'S A BRAND—NEW IDENTITY; YOU NOW BELONG TO THE PARENT CLUB.

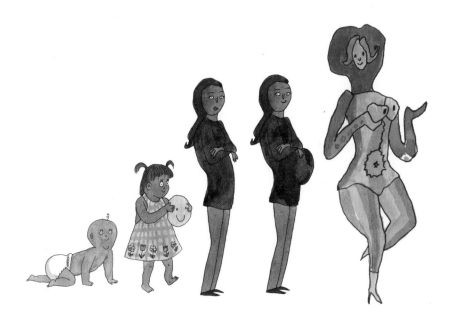

BY BECOMING A MOM, YOU WILL BECOME STRONGER, YOU WILL BE PUSHED TO YOUR LIMITS, YOU'LL BE MORE PATIENT, MORE CARING, MORE RAGEFUL THAN YOU EVER THOUGHT POSSIBLE. BEING A MOM IS HARD WORK, MUCH HARDER THAN ANYONE EVER TALKS ABOUT.

Replicating The WOMB

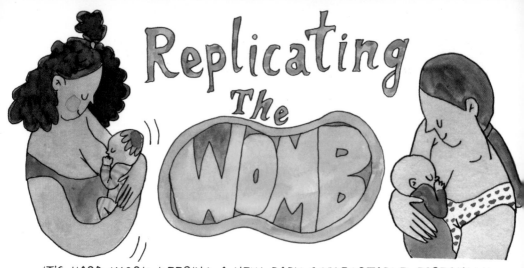

IT'S HARD WORK KEEPING A NEW BABY COMFORTABLE, ESPECIALLY DURING THE FIRST THREE MONTHS. DURING THIS TIME, BABY IS GETTING USED TO NOT BEING INSIDE ANYMORE. THINKING ABOUT WHERE BABY HAS BEEN FOR THE PAST NINE MONTHS (AKA HIS ENTIRE LIFE) CAN HELP A NEW PARENT THINK ABOUT HOW TO SOOTHE THEIR NEWBORN.

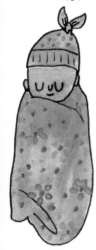

EATING OFTEN: IN THE WOMB, MOM IS CONSTANTLY NOURISHING BABY WITH NUTRIENTS THAT PASS THROUGH HER BLOOD TO THE PLACENTA AND THEN TO BABY.

LIKES TO BE ROCKED: IN THE WOMB, BABY IS CONSTANTLY MOVING BECAUSE MOMMY IS MOVING AROUND.

SWADDLING COMFORTS: IN THE WOMB, BABY IS CONSTANTLY SMOOSHED, ESPECIALLY TOWARDS THE END!

SHUSHING: IN THE WOMB, BABY IS CONSTANTLY HEARING SHUSHING SOUNDS FROM THE UTERINE LIQUIDS SURROUNDING BABY.

HOLDING: IN THE WOMB, BABY IS CONSTANTLY BEING "HELD" AND HE OR SHE IS KEPT AT THE PERFECT WARM TEMPERATURE.

Newborns

WHAT DO THEY DO?

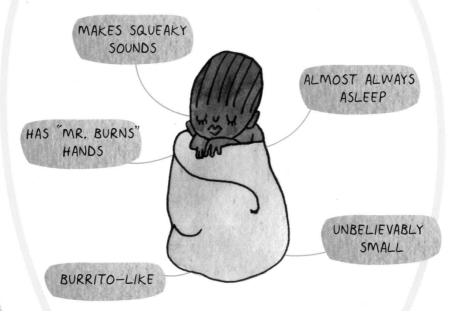

MAKES SQUEAKY SOUNDS

ALMOST ALWAYS ASLEEP

HAS "MR. BURNS" HANDS

UNBELIEVABLY SMALL

BURRITO-LIKE

THEY MAY EAT MULTIPLE TIMES AN HOUR, POOP EVERY COUPLE HOURS, AND HAVE TROUBLE LATCHING. HOWEVER, THEY ARE A JOY TO HOLD AND SNUGGLE WITH. SO SOFT AND SMALL. AND THEY EVEN HAVE THAT "NEW BABY" SMELL.

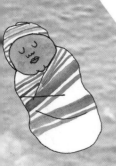

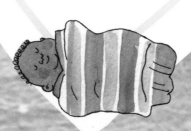

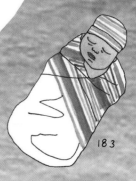

EASY WAY TO SWADDLE

1) FOLD TOP CORNER DOWN, PLACE BABY ON TOP.

2) FOLD ONE SIDE OVER BABY.

3) PULL THE BOTTOM PART UP TOWARDS BABY'S SHOULDER.

5) TUCK THAT FINAL CORNER IN.

4) TUCK THAT CORNER IN AND THEN FOLD THE OTHER SIDE OVER.

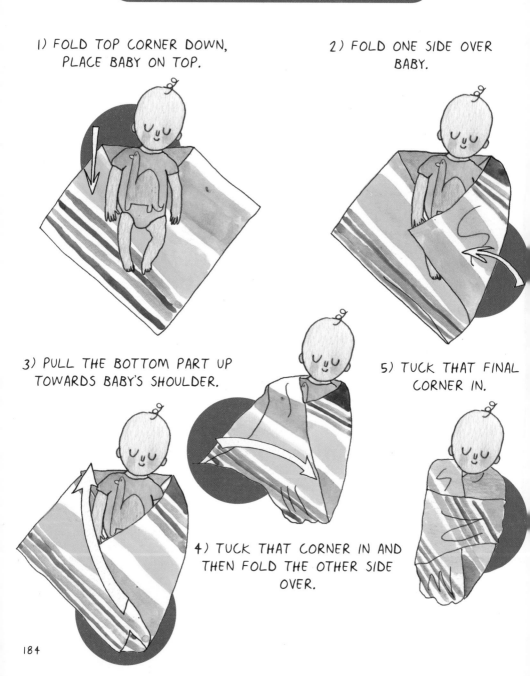

FIRST FEW WEEKS

WHEN YOU FIRST BRING BABY HOME, HE IS EATING 2—3 TIMES
AN HOUR, INCLUDING DURING THE NIGHT. IT REMINDS YOU OF ALL
THOSE "WELL INTENTIONED" PEOPLE TELLING YOU TO SLEEP
WHILE YOU WERE PREGNANT.

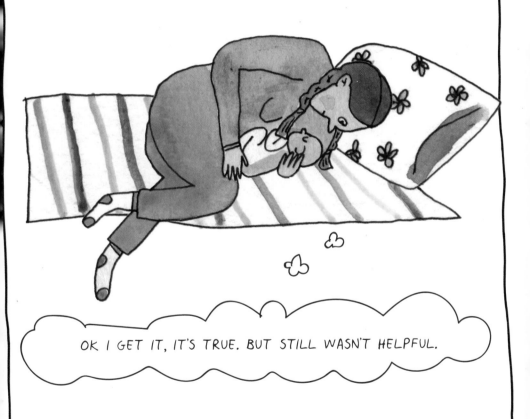

OK I GET IT, IT'S TRUE. BUT STILL WASN'T HELPFUL.

CLUSTER

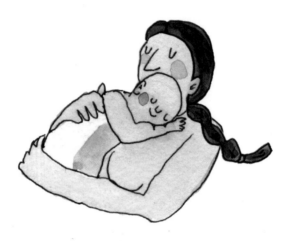

YOU ARE CONFUSED BECAUSE EVERYTHING YOU READ SAID THAT HE WOULD EAT EVERY 2-3 HOURS. YOU DID READ ABOUT CLUSTER FEEDING, WHICH MEANS THEY FEED A LOT MORE OFTEN THAN NORMAL. ONLINE, IT SAYS THAT CLUSTER FEEDING IS SUPPOSED TO HAPPEN DURING KEY MOMENTS OF DEVELOPMENT, AT CERTAIN WEEKS. IT FEELS LIKE A JOKE, BECAUSE HE HAS BEEN CLUSTER FEEDING SINCE YOU GOT HOME, AND IT DOESN'T FEEL LIKE IT'LL EVER END.

HOWEVER PAINFUL IT IS TO STAY UP
ALL NIGHT, WITH EACH FEEDING YOU
ARE DOSED WITH A HEALTHY PORTION
OF OXYTOCIN, THE BONDING AND
LOVE HORMONE.

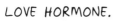

AND EVEN THOUGH YOU COULD
DRIVE YOURSELF CRAZY
THINKING ABOUT HOW LITTLE
SLEEP YOU'RE GETTING, YOU
DECIDE TO TREAT THESE
NIGHTS AS LITTLE SLEEPOVERS.
WHERE YOU DON'T ACTUALLY
SLEEP, AND YOU JUST HANG OUT
TOGETHER.

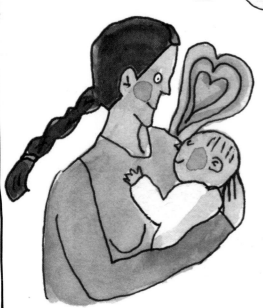

HELLO, BABY.

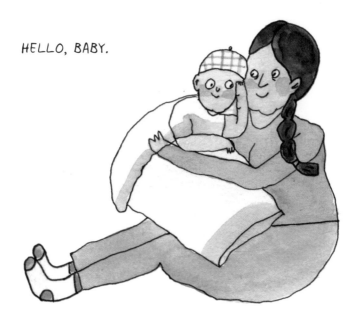

GOODBYE, SLEEP.

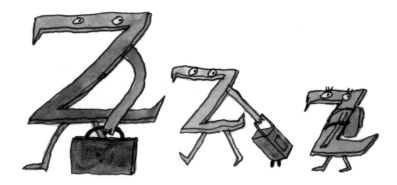

Newborn Needs

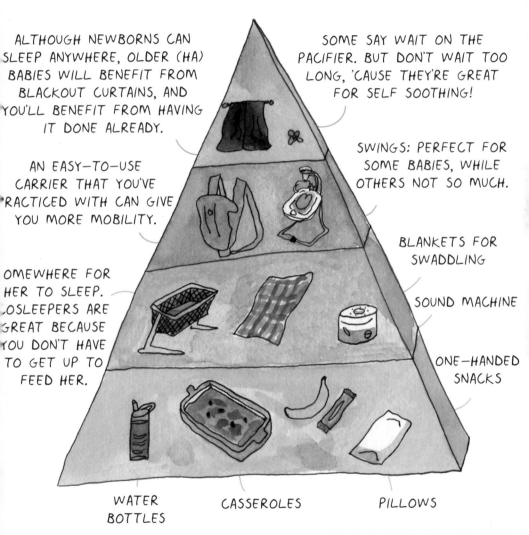

ALTHOUGH NEWBORNS CAN SLEEP ANYWHERE, OLDER (HA) BABIES WILL BENEFIT FROM BLACKOUT CURTAINS, AND YOU'LL BENEFIT FROM HAVING IT DONE ALREADY.

AN EASY-TO-USE CARRIER THAT YOU'VE PRACTICED WITH CAN GIVE YOU MORE MOBILITY.

SOMEWHERE FOR HER TO SLEEP. COSLEEPERS ARE GREAT BECAUSE YOU DON'T HAVE TO GET UP TO FEED HER.

SOME SAY WAIT ON THE PACIFIER. BUT DON'T WAIT TOO LONG, 'CAUSE THEY'RE GREAT FOR SELF SOOTHING!

SWINGS: PERFECT FOR SOME BABIES, WHILE OTHERS NOT SO MUCH.

BLANKETS FOR SWADDLING

SOUND MACHINE

ONE-HANDED SNACKS

WATER BOTTLES

CASSEROLES

PILLOWS

WHAT THE NEWBORN NEEDS MOST IS HEALTHY AND FED PARENTS, AND FOR THE PARENTS TO GET AS MUCH SLEEP AS POSSIBLE. SO WHEN PREPPING FOR NEWBORN, REMEMBER TO PREP FOR YOU!

Postpartum

BASIC ITEMS

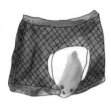

THE MESH UNDERWEAR AND BIG PADS ARE AS COMFY AS IT CAN GET, UNLESS YOU WANT TO GET ADULT DIAPERS—NO SHAME IN THAT. THE HOSPITAL WILL GIVE YOU SOME PADS AND UNDERWEAR, BUT YOU'LL ALSO WANT TO HAVE A STASH OF MAXIPADS AT HOME.

THE PERIBOTTLE IS YOUR FRIEND! FILL IT WITH LUKEWARM WATER AND SPRAY IT ON EVERY TIME YOU PEE. THE HOSPITAL WILL GIVE YOU A COUPLE. NO NEED TO BUY, UNLESS YOU WANT TO BE FANCY.

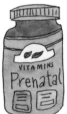

IF YOU'RE BREASTFEEDING OR PUMPING, YOU'LL WANT TO CONTINUE TO TAKE PRENATAL VITAMINS. YOU'LL ALSO WANT SOME LANOLIN ON HAND, FOR SOOTHING CHAPPED NIPS.

IF YOU'RE GOING TO BE PUMPING, AND YOUR PUMP IS NOT HANDS FREE, INVESTING IN A PUMPING BRA IS WORTH IT. I DON'T KNOW WHY THE PUMPS AREN'T AUTOMATICALLY SOLD WITH THEM. DO THEY REALLY EXPECT WOMEN TO JUST SIT THERE HOLDING THE PUMP TO THEIR BOOBS?

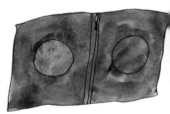

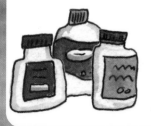

MORE PILLS! YOU WILL PROBABLY BE GIVEN ACETAMINOPHEN, STOOL SOFTENERS, AND MAYBE SOME LAXATIVES. POOPING AFTER GIVING BIRTH CAN BE DIFFICULT, AND THESE PILLS HELP WITH THAT.

AFTER YOUR 6-WEEK CHECKUP, A PHYSICAL THERAPIST APPOINTMENT POSTPARTUM SHOULD BE A NORMAL STEP OF THE PROCESS FOR EVERY NEW MOM. THERE IS A LOT OF STRETCHING THAT NEEDS TO HAPPEN TO HOLD A BABY IN THERE AND THEN PUSH ONE OUT. A P.T. CAN CHECK YOUR LADY PARTS OUT TO MAKE SURE EVERYTHING IS HEALING PROPERLY. THEY'LL ALSO GIVE YOU PERSONALIZED EXERCISES TAILORED TO YOUR NEEDS AND TEACH YOU HOW TO PROPERLY RELAX AND KEGEL.

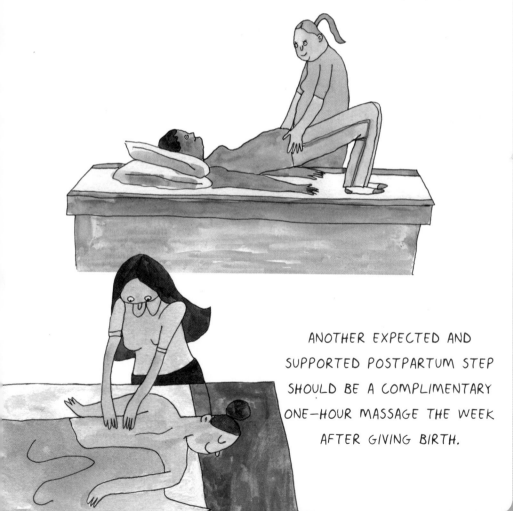

ANOTHER EXPECTED AND SUPPORTED POSTPARTUM STEP SHOULD BE A COMPLIMENTARY ONE-HOUR MASSAGE THE WEEK AFTER GIVING BIRTH.

BONDING WITH BABY

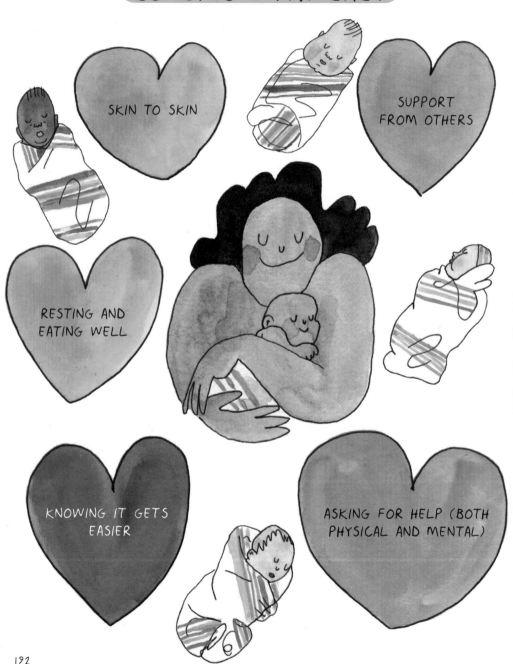

SKIN TO SKIN

SUPPORT FROM OTHERS

RESTING AND EATING WELL

KNOWING IT GETS EASIER

ASKING FOR HELP (BOTH PHYSICAL AND MENTAL)

EVERYONE IS SLEEPING BUT ME

ONE NIGHT (EVERY NIGHT?) IT SEEMS LIKE YOU ARE BREASTFEEDING EVERY HOUR AND YOU'RE THE ONLY ONE AWAKE. IT'S TOTALLY UNFAIR BECAUSE YOU ARE ALSO SO PHYSICALLY TIRED FROM BIRTH AND YOU AREN'T GETTING A BREAK OR REST. YOUR BACK, NECK, WRISTS, AND NIPPLES ALL HURT. IT'S REALLY HARD WORK BEING A MOM TO A NEWBORN, BUT YOU ARE COMFORTED BY THE REALIZATION THAT IT WON'T LAST FOREVER, BECAUSE REALLY, IT JUST CAN'T.

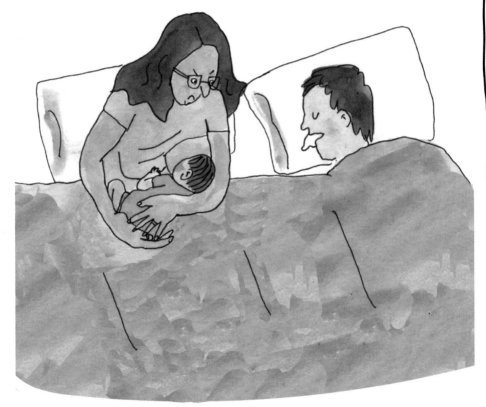

Breastfeeding

THERE ARE ENTIRE BOOKS ON THE SUBJECT,
BUT HERE ARE A FEW TIPS:

A NEWBORN'S STOMACH IS TINY!
DAY 1: 1–1.5 TEASPOONS (5–7 ML)
DAY 3: 1.5–2 TABLESPOONS (22–27 ML)
DAY 7: 1.5–2 OZ (45–60 ML)
1 MONTH OLD: 3–5 OZ (80–150 ML)

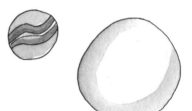

BE GENTLE ON YOURSELF. IF IT HURTS, IT COULD LEAD TO CHAPPED
NIPPLES, WHICH CAN MAKE BREASTFEEDING EVEN HARDER, SO TRY TO BE
EASY ON YOURSELF AND GIVE YOURSELF BREAKS. IT'S GOOD TO KEEP IN
MIND THAT THE BABY ONLY NEEDS SO MUCH MILK.

AFTER YOU GET THE HANG OF IT A BIT, TRY TO TAKE THAT EXTRA
MINUTE TO GET COMFY BEFORE NURSING—YOUR BACK, NECK, AND
SHOULDERS WILL THANK YOU LATER.

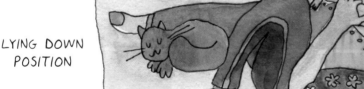

LYING DOWN
POSITION

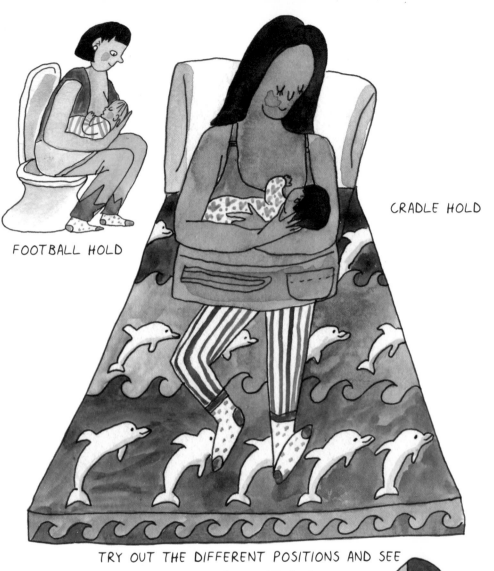

FOOTBALL HOLD

CRADLE HOLD

TRY OUT THE DIFFERENT POSITIONS AND SEE
WHICH WORK BEST FOR YOU.

LAID BACK POSITION

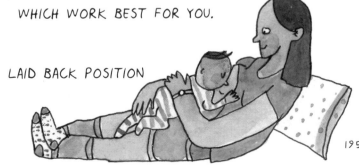

195

BREASTFEEDING CAN BE DIFFICULT

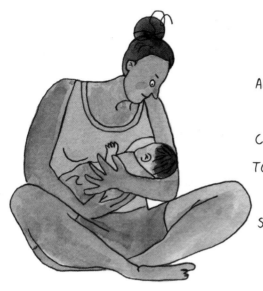

SOME HOSPITALS WILL HAVE LACTATION CONSULTANTS. TAKE FULL ADVANTAGE! LA LECHE LEAGUE IS ALSO A GREAT RESOURCE. NIPPLE SHIELDS CAN BE USEFUL IF YOU'RE STRUGGLING TO LATCH OR HAVE SORE NIPPLES, BUT CAN BE DIFFICULT TO STOP USING. SOME BABIES PREFER ONE BOOB OVER THE OTHER, SOME BABIES LIKE BOTTLES, SOME BITE....

EVEN THOUGH IT'S SO SO SO SO SO MUCH WORK, BREASTFEEDING IS A MAGICAL GIFT YOU GIVE TO YOUR BABY. IT CAN BE WORTH THE STRUGGLE OR THE ENDLESS PUMPING SESSIONS. HOWEVER, THERE IS NO MOM GUILT IN THIS BOOK. SOMETIMES FORMULA IS WHAT WORKS BEST FOR YOU AND YOUR BABY.

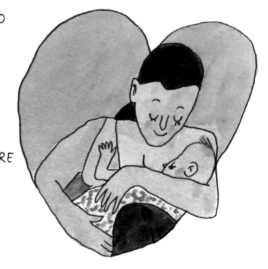

No Mom Guilt

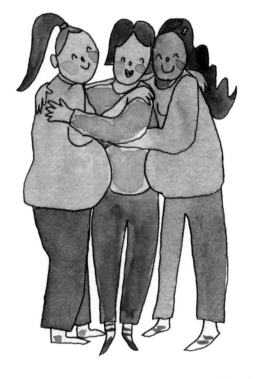

BREASTFEEDING IS ONLY ONE OF MANY THINGS THAT NEW MOMS MIGHT FEEL GUILTY ABOUT, BUT IN AN EFFORT NOT TO PERPETUATE MOM GUILT, I WON'T ATTEMPT TO LIST ANY MORE HERE. WHAT WILL BE SAID IS, YOU'RE DOING A GREAT JOB. YOUR BABY NEEDS YOU, AND YOU ARE ENOUGH. WHATEVER YOU ARE DOING IS WHAT WORKS FOR YOU AND YOUR BABY. THE REALITY IS, YOU'RE DOING A MILLION NEW THINGS WHILE SLEEP DEPRIVED. OF COURSE YOU AREN'T GOING TO DO THEM ALL PERFECTLY. THAT'S OK. IN FACT, IT'S BETTER THAN OK, BECAUSE YOU ARE LITERALLY KEEPING A BABY (WHO LEGIT IS DEPENDENT AF) ALIVE. GREAT JOB, MAMA!!!

Postpartum Depression

SPEAKING OF GUILT, SOME NEGATIVE THOUGHTS ARE NORMAL AFTER BABY COMES (AND EVEN SOMETIMES BEFORE). HOWEVER, SOME NEW MOMS AND NONBIRTHING PARTNERS CAN EXPERIENCE INTENSE NEGATIVE EMOTIONS THAT LAST FOR WEEKS OR LONGER. SINCE POSTPARTUM DEPRESSION IS SORT OF COMMON (SOME SAY UP TO 15% OF NEW MOMS EXPERIENCE IT), IT'S IMPORTANT THAT EVERYONE LEARN ABOUT THE SYMPTOMS EARLY ON.

- CRYING
- FATIGUE
- DEPRESSION
- RESTLESSNESS
- INSOMNIA
- LOSS OF APPETITE
- INTENSE IRRITABILITY
- DIFFICULTY BONDING WITH BABY

WHEN YOU'RE IN THE MIDDLE OF THE DARKNESS, IT'S DIFFICULT TO PULL YOURSELF OUT. THIS IS WHY HAVING A CLOSE PERSON WHO YOU TRUST LOOKING OUT FOR SYMPTOMS IS SO IMPORTANT. THEY CAN ADVOCATE FOR YOU AND HELP YOU GET BETTER FROM PPD, AND OTHER CONDITIONS LIKE IT, FASTER THAN YOU MIGHT ALONE. PPD DOESN'T HAVE ONE SOURCE. CHEMICAL, SOCIAL, AND PSYCHOLOGICAL CHANGES, AS WELL AS GENETICS, ARE ALL BELIEVED TO PLAY A PART. THE IMPORTANT THING IS, THERE IS HELP OUT THERE.

The Body

EMOTIONAL SUPPORT WITH PPD IS CRUCIAL, AND SO IS PHYSICAL SUPPORT AT HOME. IN SOME COUNTRIES, A NEW MOM IS EXPECTED TO PRACTICE "STAYING IN" AND LETTING OTHERS CARE FOR HER BEFORE THE BABY COMES—MAYBE SOMETHING TO CONSIDER MORE WIDELY IN THE USA. BECAUSE AFTER GIVING BIRTH, YOU NEED TIME TO RECOVER!

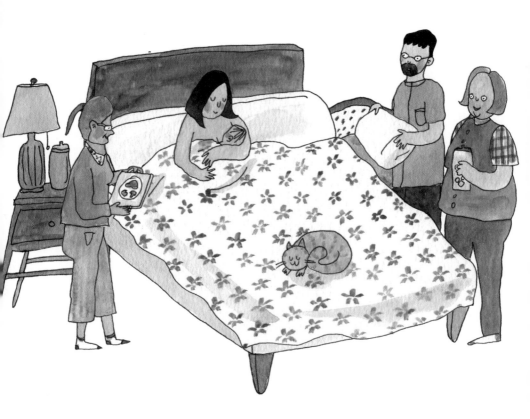

POSTPARTUM FOODS FROM AROUND THE WORLD

ALONG WITH CULTURAL TRADITIONS OF STAYING IN, LIKE "THE SITTING MONTH" IN CHINA AND "LA CUARENTENA" IN MEXICO, THERE ARE CERTAIN TRADITIONAL FOODS THAT ARE OFTEN SERVED TO POSTPARTUM MOMS. BELOW ARE SOME EXAMPLES:

VINEGAR GINGER PORK FEET SOUP

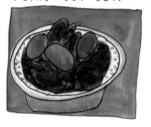

HONG KONG

CHICKEN SOUP

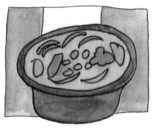

GUATEMALA

BESCHUIT MET MUISJES

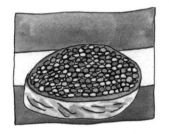

NETHERLANDS

SIMILAR TO HOW HOLIDAYS CAN BE CELEBRATED WITH SPECIAL DISHES, THESE TRADITIONAL FOODS SHOW HOW SOME CULTURES UNDERSTAND THE IMPORTANCE AND SIGNIFICANCE OF THE FIRST FEW WEEKS POSTPARTUM. IN CONTRAST, THE USA DOESN'T EVEN GUARANTEE ANY PAID TIME OFF WORK. HOPEFULLY ONE DAY WE'LL BE ABLE TO PUT MORE RESOURCES TOWARDS THIS SPECIAL TIME IN THE USA.

FINALLY,
THEY SAY WHEN YOU HAVE A BABY YOUR HEART GROWS BIGGER...

WHAT NO ONE REALLY PREPARES YOU FOR IS HOW EACH TIME
THEY OUTGROW A FAVORITE OUTFIT
OR AGE OUT OF A BED
OR HIT A BIG MILESTONE
OR...

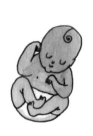

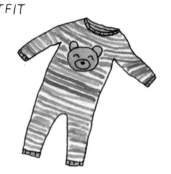

...GROW UP IN SOME SORT OF WAY, A LITTLE PART OF YOUR HEART
PAINFULLY PEELS AWAY. YOUR HEART KEEPS SHEDDING ITS SKIN SO THAT
IT CAN GROW BIGGER, TO CONTAIN THE MEMORIES OF ALL THE
DIFFERENT VERSIONS OF WHAT YOUR CHILD HAS BEEN.

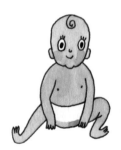

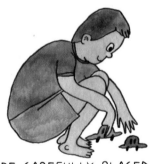

ONE DAY, YOUR BABY WILL NO LONGER NEED TO BE CAREFULLY PLACED
ON HIS BACK, OR BURPED, OR CHANGED. THESE STAGES CAN BE SO HARD,
BUT THEY SAY IT GOES BY FAST, AND IT DOES. THE GREAT THING IS,
YOU'RE JUST AT THE BEGINNING, AND YOU'RE IN FOR A WONDERFUL,
WILD RIDE. LUCKY YOU.

Thank You

I IMAGINE THIS BOOK WAS CREATED WITH ME IN A CANOE AND OTHERS COMING BY AND GIVING ME A PUSH FORWARD. IT WOULD BE TOO LONG TO GO INTO EACH PUSH, BUT I WOULD BET EVERYONE I KNOW HAS INSPIRED ME—EVEN THE MEAN ONES!

HOWEVER, I'D LIKE TO FIRST THANK MY PARENTS. MY MOM FOR ALWAYS SUPPORTING MY ART—SHE'S MY BIGGEST CHEERLEADER, AND WITHOUT HER I WOULD NEVER HAVE KEPT DRAWING. MY DAD FOR GIVING ME THE CREATIVE GENE, AS WELL AS, AND MAYBE MORE IMPORTANT, THE ABILITY TO CONFRONT AND SHARE (WHAT I BELIEVE TO BE) THE TRUTH.

I'D LIKE TO THANK MY PARTNER, MICHAEL, FIRST OFF FOR BELIEVING IN ME EVEN THROUGH HARD TIMES, AND ALSO FOR GETTING ME PREGNANT SO THIS BOOK COULD HAPPEN.

I'D LIKE TO THANK THE FRIENDS WHO READ MY BABY SHOWER BOOKLET WITH GLEE. TO ALEIA FOR ALWAYS INSPIRING ME WITH HER ART. TO LIANA FOR OPENING THE DOOR FOR ME. TO EMMA AND COLIN AT *THE NEW YORKER* FOR GIVING ME A CHANCE. TO IRVING, WHO INTRODUCED ME TO MY WONDERFUL AGENT, DANIELLE, WHO I'D ALSO LIKE TO THANK. AND, FINALLY, TO MY EDITOR, EMMA. THANK YOU.

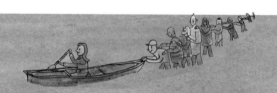

Sources

Callahan, Alice. "How Realistic Is Your Due Date?" *New York Times*, April 17, 2020. https://www.nytimes.com/2020/04/17 /parenting/due-date-accurate.amp.html.

Cooper, Erinna. "Doulas and Midwives: How Each Can Help You Have the Birthing Experience You Want." Brattleboro Memorial Hospital, January 22, 2018. https://www .bmhvt.org/doulas-midwives-can-help -birthing-experience-want.

Dekker, Rebecca. "The Evidence on: Due Dates." Evidence Based Birth, February 25, 2020. https://evidencebasedbirth.com /evidence-on-due-dates/.

Editors, The Bump. The Bump Birth Plan Tool. The Bump.com, August 19, 2014, updated January 2021. https://www.thebump.com/a /tool-birth-plan.

"Fetal Viability." Wikipedia. Wikimedia Foundation, accessed January 6, 2021. https://en.m.wikipedia.org/wiki/Fetal_viability #Medical_viability.

Gray, Caron J. and Meaghan M. Shanahan, "Breech Presentation." StatPearls [Internet], U.S. National Library of Medicine, August 11, 2020. https://www.ncbi.nlm.nih.gov/books /NBK448063/.

"Group B Strep (GBS)." Centers for Disease Control and Prevention, June 11, 2020. https://www.cdc.gov/groupbstrep /about/fast-facts.html#:~:text=About 1in 4 pregnant,onset GBS disease in newborns.

Gunter, Jen. "Massaging Away a Potential Complication of Birth?" *New York Times*, January 31, 2019. https://www.nytimes .com/2019/01/31/well/live/massaging-away -a-potential-complication-of-birth.html.

Horowitz, Evan. "Get Ready. Your Baby Is Coming Early." *Boston Globe*, July 17, 2014. https://www.bostonglobe.com/lifestyle /2014/07/17/get-ready-your-baby-coming -early/uFmISAFA2miZbw2N1c5BJJ/story.html.

Hunter, Linda A. "Issues in Pregnancy Dating: Revisiting the Evidence." *Medscape*, June 18, 2009. https://www.medscape.com /viewarticle/703501_2.

"Information About Miscarriage and Pregnancy Loss," The Miscarriage Association, accessed June 19, 2019. https://www.miscarriage association.org.uk/information/.

Karp, Harvey. *The Happiest Baby on the Block: The New Way to Calm Crying and Help Your Newborn Baby Sleep Longer.* Bantam Books, 2015.

Kindelan, Katie, and Dr. Najibah Rehman. "Exercise During Pregnancy Can Shorten Labor, Study Finds." ABC News, March 23, 2018. https://abcnews.go.com/GMA /Wellness/exercise-pregnancy-shorten -labor-study-finds/story?id=53849821.

MacDorman, Marian F., and Eugene Declercq. "Trends and State Variations in Out-of-Hos pital Births in the United States, 2004–2017." *Birth* (Berkeley, Calif.). U.S. National Library of Medicine, June 2019. https://www.ncbi.nlm .nih.gov/pmc/articles/PMC6642827/.

Marcin, Ashley, and Valinda Riggins Nwadike. "Get It On and Get It... Out? Can Having Sex Induce Labor?" *Healthline Parenthood*, January 29, 2020. https://www.health line.com/health/pregnancy/sex-to-induce -labor#takeaway.

Marple, Kate. "Growth Chart: Fetal Length and Weight, Week by Week." BabyCenter, n.d. https://www.babycenter.com/pregnancy /your-body/growth-chart-fetal-length-and -weight-week-by-week_1290794.

Martin, Joyce, Patrick Drake, Anne Driscoll, Michelle Osterman, and Brady Hamilton. "Births: Final Data for 2016," National Vital Statistics Reports. Vol. 67, Number 1. Centers for Disease Control and Prevention, 2018.

Mayo Clinic Staff. "Postpartum Depression." Mayo Foundation for Medical Education and Research, September 1, 2018. https://www.mayoclinic.org/diseases-conditions/postpartum-depression/symptoms-causes/syc-20376617.

———— . "Pregnancy Weight Gain: What's Healthy?" Mayo Foundation for Medical Education and Research, January 4, 2020. https://www.mayoclinic.org/healthy-lifestyle/pregnancy-week-by-week/in-depth/pregnancy-weight-gain/art-20044360.

"Midwife." Wikipedia. Wikimedia Foundation, accessed January 26, 2021. https://en.wikipedia.org/wiki/Midwife.

"Mizuko Kuyō." Wikipedia. Wikimedia Foundation, accessed December 31, 2020. https://en.wikipedia.org/wiki/Mizuko_kuy%C5%8D.

"Placenta." Wikipedia. Wikimedia Foundation, accessed March 2, 2021. https://en.wikipedia.org/wiki/Placenta.

"Preterm Birth." Centers for Disease Control and Prevention, October 30, 2020. https://www.cdc.gov/reproductivehealth/maternalinfanthealth/pretermbirth.html.

Reilly, Kathleen M. "Inducing Labor: Why It's Necessary and How It Works." *Parents*, June 11, 2015. https://www.parents.com/pregnancy/giving-birth/preparing-for-labor/health-101-inducing-labor/.

Richmond, David. "Perineal Tearing Is a National Issue We Must Address." Royal College of Obstetricians & Gynaecologists, July 11, 2014. https://www.rcog.org.uk/en/blog/perineal-tearing-is-a-national-issue-we-must-address/.

Ries, Julia. "I Drank Over the Holiday and Now I'm Pregnant. Is My Baby Okay?" *Family Education*, July 9, 2018, updated February 12, 2020. https://www.familyeducation.com/alcohol-during-pregnancy/i-drank-over-the-holiday-and-now-im-pregnant-is-my-baby-okay.

Roman, Ashley S. "Is It True Pregnant Women Shouldn't Take Baths?" TheBump.com, August 19, 2014, updated December 18, 2018. https://www.thebump.com/a/pregnant-women-should-not-take-baths.

Smith, Lori. "What Can Go Wrong with the Placenta during Pregnancy?" *Medical News Today*. MediLexicon International, June 15, 2018. https://www.medicalnewstoday.com/articles/309618.

Taylor, Marygrace. "Is It Normal to Have Watery Discharge During Pregnancy?" Edited by Mark Payson. WhattoExpect.com, June 4, 2020. https://www.whattoexpect.com/pregnancy/your-health/watery-discharge-during-pregnancy/.

"Thursday Tip: Newborns Have Small Stomachs!" La Leche League Canada, May 21, 2015. https://www.lllc.-ca/thursday-tip-newborns-have-small-stomachs.

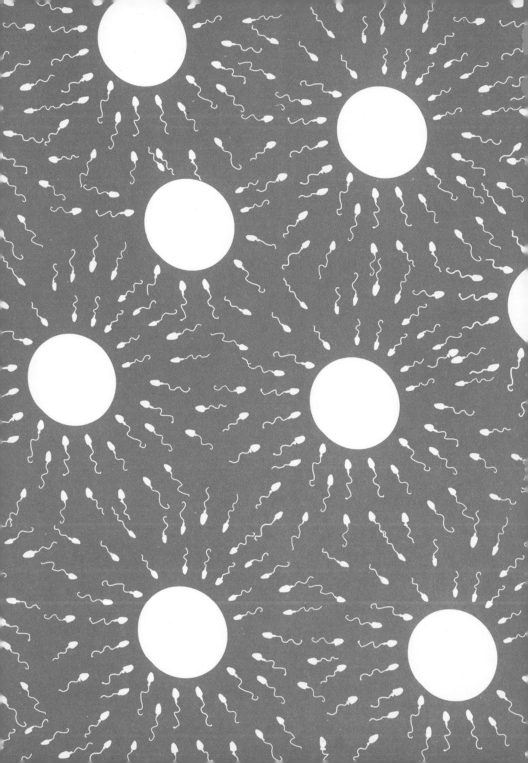